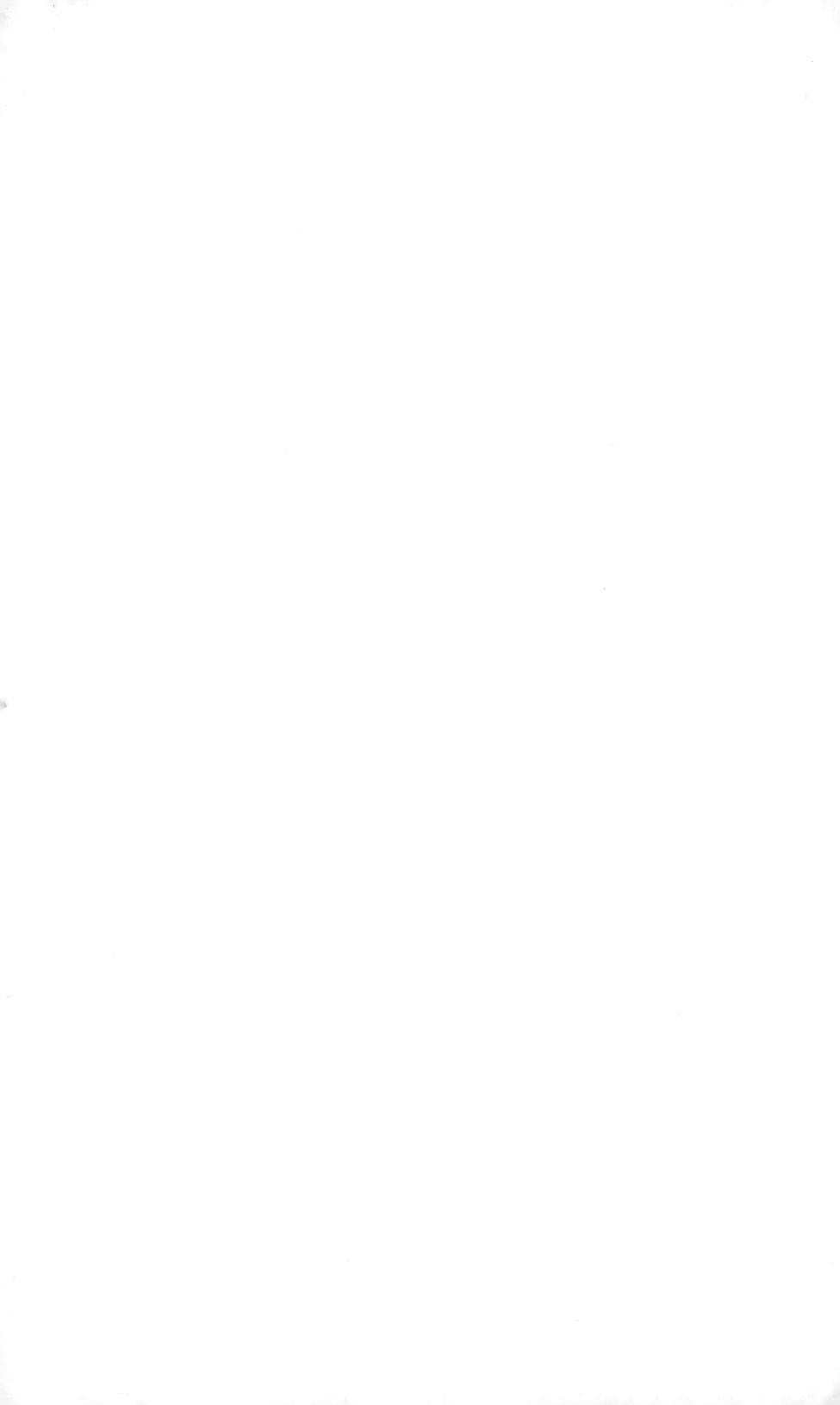

SOUL-FIT

Secrets to Living Your Best Life

JP Roche

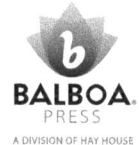

BALBOA
PRESS
A DIVISION OF HAY HOUSE

Balboa Press books may be ordered through booksellers or by contacting:

Balboa Press
A Division of Hay House
1663 Liberty Drive
Bloomington, IN 47403
www.balboapress.com
1 (877) 407-4847

Because of the dynamic nature of the Internet, any web addresses or
links contained in this book may have changed since publication and
may no longer be valid. The views expressed in this work are solely those
of the author and do not necessarily reflect the views of the publisher,
and the publisher hereby disclaims any responsibility for them.

The author of this book does not dispense medical advice or prescribe the use
of any technique as a form of treatment for physical, emotional, or medical
problems without the advice of a physician, either directly or indirectly. The
intent of the author is only to offer information of a general nature to help
you in your quest for emotional and spiritual well-being. In the event you use
any of the information in this book for yourself, which is your constitutional
right, the author and the publisher assume no responsibility for your actions.

Any people depicted in stock imagery provided by Getty Images are
models, and such images are being used for illustrative purposes only.
Certain stock imagery © Getty Images.

Print information available on the last page.

ISBN: 978-1-9822-2378-6 (sc)
ISBN: 978-1-9822-2380-9 (hc)
ISBN: 978-1-9822-2379-3 (e)

Library of Congress Control Number: 2019903207

Balboa Press rev. date: 03/15/2019

2nd May 2019.

For Fintan, truly my greatest inspiration. Thanks for shining your light so brightly. Keep going, Son!

To Niamh & Jasper,

Hope you like JP's Book, ?
it's a positive Read!

Love, from us.!
Aunty Geraldine, & young Fintan.
Much love xx

Contents

Introduction

At the heart of human desire is the desire for happiness. Whatever happiness looks like for you, you are moving towards it. One would hope that from the time of being born to that moment when you leave your body, some traction has been made. You would hope that some lessons have been learned, that some lives have been changed for the better, that some kindness and compassion have taken place, and that overall your life was a productive and happy one.

What is life all about? I believe we are all on different paths and that we have different journeys. Whatever yours may be, you have a difference to make in this lifetime, however small that difference might be. Of course we are not all kings, queens, Kardashians, or Beckhams (what a boring world it would be if such were the case!), but let's not forget that we are all born equal. We each have a divine birthright to be happy, to have success, and to experience love.

That's right, we are all born equal, and within each of us lies great potential. Some of us are great musicians. Others are brilliant at acting. There are those of us who are great at counselling others, some who are brilliant with animals and nature, those who were born to teach kids, and so on. I am always envious of those people who sort of know their purpose from a young age. It makes things as they grow up a little easier, and such people find it easier to avoid distraction. If you really know what you want to do, it makes for more straightforward decision-making. For most of us, though, it's not so clear-cut, and often it takes plenty of *living* to get to our truth.

As we become truer to ourselves, we shine our light more brightly into the world. So to answer the question "What is life all about?"— well, I'm not sure. Of course, like you, I'm just here trying to be the best me that I can be. But if I had to table an answer, it would be along the lines of becoming your most authentic self in this lifetime, warts an' all.

You see, your biggest challenge, the most hardened competitor that you will ever have to face, is you yourself. Your biggest challenge is that of overcoming the obstacles within. The world can be a scary place, but it's your perception of it that makes it either scary, safe, or beautiful. You are the one who knows yourself better than anyone else; you are the one who can talk yourself into or out of anything that is possibly conceivable in your own conscious reality. As Henry Ford once said, whether you believe you can do something or can't do something, either way you will be correct.

Your relationship with yourself, however selfish this might sound, is the most important relationship you have, and it's fundamental to uncovering your truth and finding the eternal happiness that you deserve. If you can't love and respect yourself, then what chance do you have? Not only that, but what chance does humanity have? Clearly, as a global collective, we need to make changes to enable a safe evolution for ourselves as a race and to ensure the survival of the planet. This change starts with one person, within you. The more we try to change each other and the world around us, well … Just take a look at the news and the global issues we face. That approach is a proven nonstarter.

So are you prepared to take this journey within?

If so, read on. I don't have any five-step, twenty-one-step, eight-month, or three-step processes for you. I don't have a magic pill for you to take or a combination of products to sell you once you finish reading *Soul-Fit*. Neither am I asking you to join any clubs, cults, or Facebook groups. What I offer is an honest look into the world of mindful practice and something I call "soul fitness". We talk a lot about mind, body, and soul. Finding a balance between all three is one of the keys to living a healthy, balanced, and happy life.

It's pretty easy to relate to and understand the concepts of body and mind, but do you really understand what the soul element involves? Maybe you do personally, but for us as a society it's certainly not something that we speak much about or that is high on any agendas. Given its importance, I find that crazy. Of the three elements, the soul is, in my opinion, the most profound, powerful, and successful at eliciting positive change.

I'm not a conspiracy theorist either, by the way. I could argue that the powers that be have purposely kept the education curriculums archaic for a reason, have purposely held back from us key information about the workings of the human experience, and have, by using divide-and-conquer tactics through proxy wars across the globe, fooled us into living a life fuelled by fear. I think that these powers, by using a fractional reserve banking system, have made it so that a very small number of people become rich whilst most learn only how to keep their heads above water, forgetting that we all are equal.

No, I'm not going to get into any of that. What I will do, though, is take you through a journey of the internal experience, a journey of the soul and all its workings, so that you can make informed decisions about your conscious experience. Take your time as you read through *Soul-Fit*. Let it soak in, and keep an open mind. The aim here is for you to find your truth, not anybody else's. Herein lies ancient wisdoms and secrets that will help you unlock your great potential and live your best life.

You deserve it. Go make it happen, whatever it is.

Note: Soul-Fit is set out in three parts. Part 1 looks at the essence of being a human in this turbulent modern world. In part 2 we take a deep dive into the techniques, wisdoms, and practices that can help you find your most authentic self. Part 3 wraps it all up and will help you achieve greater understanding, grounding, and balance. I have not written *Soul-Fit* for you to read in any particular way. You may read it in any way that you see fit. My objectives in writing *Soul-Fit* are to give a better understanding of the soul element of a human being, to promote meditation as a daily activity, and to help any person looking for help in even the smallest way. I've written the words that follow from my heart to yours. Please read them in the same spirit of compassion and kindness.

1

Part

IDENTITY

I believe that the very purpose of our life is to seek happiness. That is clear. Whether one believes in religion or not, whether one believes in this religion or that religion, we are all seeking something better in life. So, I think, the very motion of our life is towards happiness.

—Dalai Lama

So we are all moving in a general direction, and that direction is towards happiness. Happiness can mean many things. It's a general term that we might use to describe a sense of well-being, contentment, and balance. We may derive happiness from material things, those objects that having wealth can offer, such as nice cars and a big home. Nice cars, homes, objects, and material things are all "nice" according to one's opinion.

Maybe it's inner peace that you are after. Hopefully after reading *Soul-Fit*, you will have a better sense of what inner peace means and how to attain it. What's clear is that happiness means many things to many different people and that there is more to this world than a material realm. In addition to the material realm that we see, hear, touch, and smell, there is a spiritual realm that is intertwined with it. One is born out of the other. Indeed, neither can exist without the other, so a true sense of happiness should involve both.

A balance is necessary between your internal and external worlds to achieve happiness. If you only strive for material gain, you would so at the cost of your spiritual well-being. Conversely, if all you do is pray, you'll be missing out on the glory of life, all the riches it has to offer.

Happiness involves feelings, and feelings are very much on the inside. When we say "happy," we are describing a feeling, so happiness is an internal entity, a vibration. Learning to cultivate it is the motion of life that the Dalai Lama talks about. Move in the direction that makes you happiest. Move within your authentic nature, and be comfortable in your own skin. Happiness, then, is not just the material gains or just a high we experience sometimes from the acquisition of material objects. True happiness is a journey. Learning to appreciate that journey is the key to cultivating your true wealth and nature. Extremes or false highs should be avoided if one is to experience true happiness and eternal joy.

You are a human being. So am I. It's pretty simple. We could take some advice from our friends in the animal kingdom who see each other as equals. There's no "your house is bigger than my house" or similar ego-driven judgements, just simply, "I am a dog and you are a dog, so let's bark!" There may be animal instincts and a survival nature amongst animals, but animals are very much in the moment, creatures that live in the *now*, more often than we are. How do I know that? Well, have you ever seen a cat wearing a watch?

As a human, are you living in the moment? How much judging are you doing? Are you concerned with what other human beings think of you based on your illusory labels?

Illusory Labels

We assign many labels to ourselves. There is a whole curriculum vitae of who you think you are. Interestingly, if I were to look back at all the CVs I have written over the years, I would discover that I have changed a lot. The CV I wrote about twenty years ago is nothing like the one I would write now if I needed to. It would be almost as if I were describing two completely different people who happened to have the same name. What does this tell you? That many of your labels and the ID that you present to the world changes a lot as you go through life, but essentially the truth within, your soul, the real you, never changes. It's just that this bit doesn't go on anyone's CV. Can you imagine, just below your contact details and then your bio, a new heading, "My Soul Mission"?! What would you write?

So rather than "Jo Bloggs, British citizen, *x* years old, married to Sarah, degree in business studies, works as a banker," it would be, "Jo Bloggs, human being, lives on planet Earth, soul mission as yet unknown, but having loads of fun finding out and letting go of the other labels that don't really define my truth and eternal nature."

Of course we need labels; we need ego. In order to define ourselves and recognise each other, we use ego and labels. However, the downside to overidentifying with our labels is that it puts us in competition with each other. We worry about what others think. We lose sight of soul value and focus only on external material things. Know that labels are also outside of you, so the more you identify with them, the more lost you become, and potentially the more unhappy deep down you will become.

The more we see each other as competition, the more we are identifying with the ego self. It's easy to see how this happens. Have you ever seen a black baby and a white baby judge each other or not want to embrace each other based on their skin colour? Things like racism and negative judgement of each other are learnt and become unconscious acts. We start at school, where we learn to be in competition from an early age. Likely we get segmented into classes based on test results, so you'll see a class of pupils who know they are clever and then other students who get judged on an assessments and are put in a group that is perceived as less intelligent. Who makes these tests? They are unfair. How can intelligence be based on a math and English test? There are so many forms of intelligence.

From here it spreads. Continuing down this path, we get into not just "my class is better than your class" but also "my school is better than your school." My house is bigger than your house. My dad drives a better car than yours does. My skin colour is better than your skin colour. My race is better than yours. North London vs. South London; Northern Ireland vs. Southern Ireland; Scotland, England, and Wales. Come to think of it, how many nations don't have regional differences and judgements based simply on their geographical location? And don't get me started on religion!

When you boil it down to its component parts, you see that this type of competition and judgement is simply ridiculous. And it needs to stop. How? Don't try to change the world; you'll do that by just changing yourself, as we are all intricately connected at the subatomic level. (More on quantum mechanics coming up.) It's not easy to drop all the labels and stop all the judgement, especially because it is so ingrained in our societies, but a good starting place is to become more self-reflective. Start noticing when you are making negative judgements of others. When you do, analyse what you're doing it and see if you can change your perceptions to a more kind and compassionate viewpoint.

Look at it this way: Think of someone you don't like. You may *hate* this person. Perhaps it's someone at work whom you always go out of your way to avoid. Every time this individual speaks, you just cringe, and often confrontations with this person leave you feeling riled and angry.

Now imagine you are walking past a house that is burning. You have a flash of inspiration to help as you can see someone struggling to break a window and get out. When you get closer, you see that it's that person, your nemesis! You are in the heat of the moment—really it's your subconscious that is in control—and without hesitation you smash the window with a brick and you help the person out. Afterwards the two of you speak and the person thanks you, all the past differences forgotten in an instant.

In the great scheme of things, when it all comes down to it, what really matters in life? Ask yourself.

Above all else, rather than trying to be right all the time, try showing more kindness and compassion. It is the cornerstone to dismantling your real nemesis: ego.

Ego

A man said to Gautama Buddha, "I want happiness." Buddha told him, "First remove I. That's ego. Then remove want. That's desire."

Ego is a necessary part of the human experience. In a lot of the research I have undertaken, I've found that ego normally gets a bad rap. It's because ego is that part of us that is not truly us, and by following the impetuous nature of the ego, we normally end up in a place that's not part of our soul's mission or purpose.

Don't listen to your head. Your head wants you dead!

Not to put the shockers on too much here, but your ego also wants you dead! It's not going to mask itself and come to life in the night and attack you with a dagger; it's much subtler than that. You see, your ego is that part of you, as already mentioned, that keeps you separated from others. Important as it may be to remain distinct, really we are all connected. Before we get into that, let's gain a better understanding of the part the ego plays.

We have established that ego is that part of us that keeps us separated and enables us to recognise each other. It's that part of us that has an opinion and wants to be right. From the ego come all the lower-self emotions, things like anxiety, fear, and hate. However, on the plus side, ego is what enables you to navigate through many situations in life. It is the calculating part of a human.

The ego is good for business dealing, being competitive, getting angry, single-mindedness, choosing fear over love, being right all the time (even when you may know you are wrong), lying, and other sly behaviour. If you only live by the impulses of your ego self, you may get yourself into some very hot water.

Where is your ego? Think of the classic scenario of the devil on one shoulder and an angel on the other. Guess which one represents ego?!

The internal chatter that we all experience can be driven by two forces, one being ego and the other being divine in nature. You can normally tell what is ego; it is that impetuous nature you have. Addicts know it well. Ego is the force behind addiction, something that we have probably all experienced on one level or another, whether we care to admit it or not. You don't have to be a down-and-out alcoholic to have an alcohol addiction. And just because you don't spend all your wages on shopping doesn't mean you don't have compulsive buying issues.

We all suffer from internal conditions born of the ego, and the worst one of these is overthinking. Ego is surface-level, impetuous, reactive thinking, whereas tapping into something deeper, more soul felt, takes a bit of practice. But once you start to notice the difference and thus can make more aligned decisions, you will experience more flow in your life. You can start to break the bad habits that the ego helped you to form, and you can start to break down the ego itself.

Perhaps food is a problem for you. Whatever your sabotaging nature, it is driven by ego. Ego urges you to have that extra slice of pizza because it tastes so good. But hang on, you're on a diet, right? As we learn through *Soul-Fit* some ideas and ways to make better decisions, we can learn to break down the ego.

What happens when you break the ego down completely? Living free of ego is the ultimate aim of many spiritual practices. In some sects of Buddhism it is known as the "faceless state." Faceless because the ego is your face, the illusory label that you present to the world based on you current thinking. Once you are able to relinquish this, you don't become invisible; you just become more aligned with reality, with truth, with your authenticity. You become truly humble.

It may not be possible to achieve in this lifetime, but to become more aware of this internal battle, to start to make decisions based on truth and love rather than fear, is to begin to make the transition. The transition is to love. When it was written that love conquers all, well, I could probably stop writing right here because in a nutshell that's the answer to all the mysteries of the world, including the problem of the ego self. However, I have a few more secrets for you.

Love vs. Fear

> Fear knocked on the door, Love answered and there was nobody there.
>
> —Wayne Dyer

"Love thy neighbour as you love yourself." This is another quotation that hopefully I don't need to reference, seeing as it's a suggestion that has been with us for thousands of years now. Yet do any of us really follow this humble teaching?

What is fear? A bit like the ego, fear is another necessary part of the human experience. In a sense there is good fear and bad fear. You might label an adrenaline rush that prepares you for the fight-or-flight response a good thing. It's the kind of fear that could save your life after all. But how many times has your fear gotten the better of you?

When I say "gotten the better of you," I mean how many times has it stopped you from doing something that deep down you knew you should have done? Perhaps it was asking that person out on a date or asking your boss for a pay rise. Perhaps fear got in the way and prevented you from taking a chance like changing your career or saying what you felt was really true rather than just agreeing for the sake of not upsetting someone. Here we can see how fear can be a real party pooper, the party being your ultimate happiness and success, of course.

The root cause of such fear? Subconscious programming plays a big part. Somewhere deep down in many of us there is a sense of shame, for example, an embarrassment from childhood that has stuck and led to a painful need to fit in. This need to fit in is a function of the ego. I don't want to ask you to drudge up all your past hurts, and I don't need to; they are all stored perfectly in your subconscious mind. We sort of function on memories. All of life is memories replaying, really. Unless you can learn to release all these memories, they will continue to replay. I will show you in part 2 how to work on releasing these past hurts and memories.

Have you noticed how it's the same fears and issues that tend to replay? Unless you can learn the lessons that these fears offer you, they will continue to be prevalent in your life. In a sense, then, even so-called bad fear can be good. All fear gives you an opportunity to break through the fear. As we face our fears and overcome them, however insignificant, we convert a little more darkness into light.

In addition to overcoming fear and thus removing some of the internal blocks that reside within you, there are also plenty of opportunities in life to choose love over fear. How can you be more compassionate today? How can you show kindness to someone today? Don't let fear get in the way of showing more love and joy to the world, because truly that would be a tragedy.

Always remember fear like this: FEAR—false evidence appearing real. Much of life is a projection. It is a very persuasive illusion but is an illusion nonetheless. Fear is very much a part of this illusion, whilst love is the true reality that we each must strive to understand and better perceive. We project from our internal space, so if your automatic pilot is always set on a state of fear, anxiety, or worry, then you will likely attract events that cause such feelings so as to support that inner projection. Your mind is an extremely powerful tool. Many fears are just created by an overthinking and incorrectly used mind. Learn to tap into the deeper wisdom that resides within you, your soul, and thus bypass the incorrect use of the overthinking mind. When you grasp this truth, you will watch unnecessary fear slip away and will be more able to consciously choose love.

There are some major benefits to choosing love over fear too. How about supreme health and well-being for a start? Bruce Lipton is an expert on genetic biology. He explains it better than I could in the following excerpt from his book *The Biology of Belief*:

> You can choose what you see. You can filter your life with rose coloured beliefs that will help your body grow or you can use a dark filter that turns everything black and makes your body/mind more susceptible to disease. You can live a life of fear or live a life of love. You have the choice! But I can tell you that if you choose to see a world full of love, your body will respond by growing in health. If you choose to believe that you live in a dark world full of fear, your body's health will be compromised as you physiologically close yourself down in a protection response.

Subconscious Mind

Think of a projector and a screen. Perhaps you are doing a presentation using these as your method of delivery. If there is a technical issue and the presentation does not play, what do you do? Likely you will look to the computer from which the presentation is being drawn or the projector itself, but rarely will you go to the projector screen, as that's just the canvas on which the presentation plays out.

Well, why then in life do so many of us, when in the clutches of fear and perceived problems, look to change the external events through which we see the problems playing out? That is like going to the projector screen when the real issues lie within the workings of the computer or projector.

In this case the projector is you, your internal space, and much of that is determined by your subconscious mind. The subconscious mind is a wonderfully powerful entity, a storehouse of memories if you will. Your subconscious allows you to do a great many things without thinking. It allows you to multitask and just get things done. Without it, you'd still be learning how to walk, never mind perform simple tasks we all take for granted like tying your shoelaces or driving a car.

Take driving, for instance. Imagine all the data, thinking, muscular ability, nerve synapses, and so on it takes to drive a car. Not only that, but also you are bombarded with external inputs like road signs, busy traffic, and the noise of the radio. In addition to this, there are your internal goings-on, such as thinking about the future or worrying about the past. It's all happening, yet you can drive for miles without consciously doing so. There's the magic of the subconscious mind; it keeps us alive and safe.

It is said that the consciousness that you experience is only 5 per cent of the picture and that the other whopping 95 per cent is happening subconsciously and thus you are unaware of it. Can you believe that? Only 5 per cent!

The subconscious mind literally processes around two million bits of information per second, a task, I think you'll agree, that our conscious minds would not be capable of. I'm in trouble with anything more than two tasks at one time! It's the old iceberg analogy. Imagine that your conscious mind with its five senses is the tip of the iceberg, whilst what is really driving the ship and making things happen is that 95 per cent that is submerged.

You are the captain of your own ship, so where do you want to sail to? You can do anything you want to do with your life. That's the deal down here on planet Earth. Despite what you may have been taught, and definitely despite the standards that you think others and society hold you to, it's really only about you and your desires.

The best way to make things happen is by tapping into that 95 per cent, the computer, the projector, but *never* the 5 per cent, the screen or the environment in which your life plays out. Through the rest of *Soul-Fit* we look at ways of affecting this 95 per cent so you can use it to your advantage to make things happen in your life, to steer your ship in the right direction with the understanding that life is really about the journey and not about your perceived destination. If you don't know where you are going or where you want to go, that doesn't matter. As you tap into your soul and your truth, things will start to unfold for you, but first you must learn how to be yourself and, more important, how to love yourself.

The issue with the subconscious mind is that we have come to rely on it too much and we need to take back some of that 95 per cent. You see, many of us are only on autopilot and are not in any way mindful of the life we have. Habits can be good, and they can be bad. They are all formed in the subconscious mind, but we can consciously decide to change them. We can work with our subconscious mind to let go of all the memories that stem back for generations and that can still be having a negative impact on our current experiences.

In addition to your own subconscious mind, there is the universal subconsciousness. This is what enables the universe to keep ticking. It's what allows the seasons to unfold; it's how a bird knows to migrate to the other side of the planet; it's how a hedgehog knows to hibernate; and it's how your hair knows to keep growing (or not, in my case!). If your own subconscious keeps you alive by breathing for you, amongst doing billions of other things, well then, the universal subconsciousness is what keeps the universe alive and kicking and is where of all of life's serendipities stem from—the way things just work out.

You and I and all living things are connected to this divine source, and we are connected via a higher self. The higher self can be referred to as the soul. So, you see, as we learn to take back some of the 95 per cent, we connect with our deeper internal selves, connecting back to Source. The connection is energetic, not material, in the same way that your soul is energetic but not material. You can't put your hands on it, but that doesn't mean you can't affect it or work on it or, indeed, work with it.

Your subconscious mind then is the doorway to your internal experience. It is the doorway to change and the doorway to divinity if that's what you are into. Whatever your journey, the secrets to it are held within your soul, and the path to success and happiness lies within your subconscious mind, as that is the engine room of your existence. Your higher self will know the best route forward for you.

Flow

Think of a time when you have been in flow. By flow I mean you have done things effortlessly and really well. A professional sportswoman, for instance, can go about her game without much thought. She can score goals or tries or win points by thinking less. Much of this success has been learnt through practice.

By practising things, we assign them to memory, and then the subconscious mind takes over when in the throes of a game. But that's not all that is happening, because although motor movements are stored in memory, there are other factors at play. This sportswoman is also making critical decisions under duress about things that she has not learnt before. Because they are new events, they are not coming from the storehouse of memory.

When in flow, we are guided by a force greater than us. In such a situation, the more you think, the worse things can get. As you let go of your need to control and think, you move into a different type of experience where effortless flow can occur and things just fall into place. This is universal subconsciousness, and you are an integral part of it. You are worthy. There is no one on earth now, there has not been anyone on earth at any time in the history of humankind, and there is no one yet to be born who is more worthy than you are now of success and happiness. So what's stopping you?

The more you try to control things outside of yourself, the worse things will become. The only thing you can realistically change is yourself, and the way to do this is consciously through the subconscious mind. You can also look to quantum mechanics for more evidence of how things really are.

Quantum Mechanical Theory

> Our sight consists of a hypothesis, an interpretation of the world. We don't see the data in front of our eyes; we see an interpretation.
>
> —Richard Gregory

This theory has profound implications and gives new meaning to our lives as well as insight into who we really are and the landscape within which we all find ourselves here on earth. As already stated, your conscious awareness only experiences at best 5 per cent of what is really going on. To recap, this basically means two major things:

1. We, within our own realities and what we think of as the true nature of all things (conscious awareness), don't actually have a clue as to what's going on. Therefore, if we want to actually start acting as conscious cocreators of our own lives (which we have the power to be), we need to start accepting this fact by working within the true nature of reality, within the subconscious mind, which is connected to a higher power (higher consciousness or superconsciousness), which you don't necessarily need to call God although some people do.

2. We don't in reality see with our eyes. We process light through our eyes, but our interface of what we think we see is coming from the brain, specifically a process centre called the thalamus. In Eastern culture, this is the location of the chakra ashna or third eye chakra. In short, we see what we need to see to support the vibration of our inner world, which is determined, ultimately, by our thoughts, feelings, and emotions (thoughts with energy).

One way to check on your inner world, in fact the easiest and surest way, is to look at your life right now. Look at what your outer world holds for you, including all the material things. How's your job going? What are your finances like? Love life? Car? And so on. What do you see when you think of these things? What inner feelings are stirred? Do they stimulate a higher, lighter vibration of a love-based entity, or are you in a dense state of worry?

Either way, you will be correct. Whatever vibrational state you are in acts as the magnet in your life for all that you have manifested for yourself. And according to quantum theory, which states that we, the observer of our lives, create what we observe, and thus we manifest those things in our material realm concurrent with this internal state.

In his book *Understanding Quantum Thinking*, Mark Dawes goes on to explain that the reality of what we experience in our physical world depends entirely on our observation of it:

> Quantum Mechanics states that objects are created by observation of them. As a result the observer creates the reality of what exists. In other words, atoms and sub-atomic particles do not exist anywhere until they are observed. In short, everything exists in fields of unending possibilities and it is not until we observe that potential that the reality collapses in to existence. As a result there is a scientific connection between conscious observation and the material world. Today all physicists generally accept the principle that quantum theory applies universally, and if that is so, then all reality is created by observation.

What we are undergoing is a phenomenally intricate, amazing, and wonderful life experience, so intricate and boundless, in fact, that unless we can let go and let God, we don't have a hope in hell of manifesting a meaningful existence for ourselves. What quantum theory tells us is that the more we try to micromanage our lives, the more we apply our inferior thinking conscious minds directed by ego to the task of directing our lives, the more likely we are ultimately to fail or cause pain. The essence of this is that through positive thinking and spirituality, we free ourselves and enable our lives to flourish in line with all that is. Furthermore, the gifts that life has in store for us cannot be realised if we have to have things a certain way, as we might get what we wish for, but we won't get all the blessings that lay in wait and would have been ours had we not been so determined to achieve those particular outcomes. Relinquish the ego's control doesn't mean a life free of obstacles and pain, but it does mean a life directed towards those wishes and desires that we truly have, that our souls desire.

In essence, what quantum theory tells us is that everything exists in fields of unending possibilities, thus we can tap into any future reality we desire if we can tune into it correctly. The possibility you seek will collapse into reality if you do this part right. This sounds easy, but actually it takes a considerable bit of disciplined effort on your part. Yet as the Chinese proverb goes, the best time to plant a tree was twenty years ago, and the next best time is now!

> Sometimes we must undergo hardships, breakups and narcissistic wounds, which shatter the flattering image that we had of ourselves, in order to discover two truths: that we are not who we thought we were; and that the loss of a cherished pleasure is not necessarily the loss of true happiness and well-being.
>
> —Jean-Yves Leloup

Part 1 Conclusions

We are spiritual beings living a human experience and not the other way around. That which is within you is your true self, not your labels.

There are many layers to being a human being. In addition to all the energetic levels, you have a soul, a subconscious mind, and a higher self, all intricately connected.

We are all connected to each other at a subtle subatomic level, and we are all connected to the same source, whatever that means for you. For me it is the Divine Source, not something I call God but love.

The energy of love is all-powerful and all-encompassing, and you and I are an integral part of it.

There is nothing to fear, as fear is an illusion created by the ego to keep us separated from our truth.

By being more mindful, we can become more mindless. Mindfulness is a kind of brain training that can help us overcome our overthinking minds, which tend to lead us astray.

The subconscious mind is the key to change. If you want to achieve your desires, then you can reprogramme your subconscious mind to do so. I will show you how in parts 2 and 3 of *Soul-Fit*.

You can literally achieve anything you want to, but first it's best to understand who you truly are and what you truly desire.

2
Part
FIT SOUL

n this part, we will explore how to cultivate a fit soul by exercising your spiritual muscles and reprogramming your subconscious mind.

Meditation

> No retreat offers someone more quiet and relaxation than that into his own mind.
>
> —Marcus Aurelius

One of the best ways to get to the bottom of who you are is to meditate. I believe that meditation is a lost art and something that is as integral and important to a human being as water is to a fish. Without it, we starve our souls.

The tide is turning as more and more people are turning to ancient techniques and wisdoms such as meditation. We are in unprecedented times with a high number of cases of stress-related problems such as heart disease, anxiety, depression, cancer, and addiction.

These types of stress-related illnesses are on the up, so the real killer here, rather than the symptomatic illnesses themselves, is of course stress. The modern lifestyle is causing so much stress, distress, and disease. When we are out of sync with ourselves, when we are striving in the wrong way and putting this increased stress on ourselves, we should find it to be no surprise that bad things can happen with our health and our happiness.

Meditation is an antidote to this problem.

Other benefits of meditation include improved sleep, slowed brainwaves and heart rate, reduced blood pressure, the ability to overcome bad habits, and a deepening of your spiritual connection, thus bringing you closer to your soul and your true desires.

Mindfulness is another great practice that encompasses all the benefits of meditation and brings these into your everyday practices and behaviours. Mindfulness is good because it teaches us to be in the moment, in the now. You can be waiting in a queue at the bank or stuck in traffic in your car, and rather than getting stressed and damning your situation, you become mindful. A mindfulness practitioner would look for the reasons to be grateful in such a situation and might decide to do a body scan (see the following subsection) or perhaps take the opportunity to show some kindness towards another person—basically anything apart from working oneself into a frenzy.

Mindfulness and meditation are good because they are a kind of brain training. They teach you to think less, and they help train the mind to be more focused. So rather than getting caught up in your unwanted thoughts all the time (running on autopilot), you can actively direct your thoughts more efficiently towards your goals and desires (consciously cocreating).

Thinking, by the way, isn't all that good. Thoughts essentially are a bit of a problem for a productive and fruitful existence. I'm talking about the monkey mind here, the incessant internal chatter led by the ego that can tie you up in all sorts of mental knots.

As Bruce Lee once said, "Don't think. Feel." This is the essence of getting soul-fit.

The power of thought is massive. For example, remember a time when you thought you had lost your keys. The panic sets in, and suddenly you see yourself locked outside your home in the freezing cold and rain for hours on end. After a moment of calm, of mindfulness, you either find your keys at the bottom of your bag or simply get the spare set from the neighbour you left them with. Thoughts are powerful as they create your reality. This is why it's so important that you have some sway over them and use them to your advantage.

The good news is: *you are not your thoughts!*

Furthermore, *you get to decide your thoughts!*

As Mike Dooley from TUT (The Universe Talks) says, "Thoughts become things. Choose the good ones."

How do you gain more sway over your thoughts, becoming more proactive in your own life and less at the behest of your autopilot?

Meditate more!

Meditation and mindful practice are the gym tools for your brain that will enable you to get better and better at noticing your thoughts and redirecting them towards your goals, success, and happiness. If the subconscious mind is the portal to the soul, then thoughts are the portal to reprogramming the subconscious mind.

It is important to state, when talking about meditation, that there is no bad meditation. And the beauty of it is that it is very versatile.

Let's get it clear that you do not need to be a Buddhist monk to meditate. You don't need to be in the lotus position for hours on end, and you don't have to be in a quiet place to meditate, though of course this would be preferable. You can practise for five minutes or twenty in the peace and quiet of your own home, or you can practise methods of meditation in the queue at the supermarket. A little bit of meditation often is better than a few longer sessions each week. This should be a daily practice.

As you progress, you will learn through practice how to become the witness to your thoughts and to your life. The more you do this, the more able you will be in everyday life to be able to resist getting caught up in autopilot mode. Thus you refrain from fretting over the past and worrying about the future. This can be very liberating and peaceful.

As you begin to meditate, your ego at times, through your thinking, might lead you to feel a bit silly. It may tell you that you are wasting your time, that perhaps you should be doing something more productive with your time, and that the meditation isn't working. Know this is your ego. This may sound daft to you, but I guarantee it to be true: your ego self does not want you meditating!

Start slowly and build it up. Meditation is one of your best spiritual muscles, and like any physical muscle, through work and practice it will become stronger, thus making you become stronger.

Aim for three to five minutes of meditation a day if you are a beginner. Also for a beginner, a quiet place is best to avoid distractions. You don't need to be cross-legged on the floor, but if you choose to sit in a chair, remain upright with your back in its natural curved posture rather than slumped. You don't want to turn this into a power nap.

Close your eyes and focus your attention on your breathing. Imagine the air coming in through the centre of your nostrils, and follow the breath into the depth of your diaphragm. If you are good at visualising and with seeing colours in your mind's eye, then you can imagine breathing in a white stream of air and exhaling a pink stream. If this doesn't resonate with you, just focus on the breathing.

After some initial deeper breaths, start to slow your breathing down so it moves more into its normal rhythm. If any thoughts pop into your mind, just let them pass through, and if you can, do not attach to them. Don't run with them. But if you get caught out, don't worry; just bring your focus back to your breathing. Don't forget that for most of our early lives, we have just allowed ourselves, out of ignorance, to attach to our thoughts and thus become like unconscious robots. It's become habit, so don't beat yourself up if you keep thinking about what you are going to have for dinner tonight. You are now learning a new habit. Initially this can be challenging. As with learning anything new, you need repetition to get better.

For the first few times, the only thing you may do is just spend a few minutes in breathing-focused meditation. If you want to add some time, and if you feel comfortable enough, after a few minutes of breathing-focused meditation, start to bring in some of the other techniques described in the following sections. As you get better at meditating, you will find five or even ten minutes will fly by. Then you will be ready for more advanced versions of meditation.

Try this method at least two times a day, preferably in the morning and in the evening, and at any other times of the day that may be appropriate for you.

Remember, there is no bad meditation. Even if you feel your meditation wasn't good, you will undoubtedly gain something positive from it. Meditation is about respecting your inner world. And as you get more in tune with your inner world, the more healing will take place for you in your life, the better your vibration will be, and the more noticeable it will become to others that you are doing something positive in your life. You will literally be exuding positivity.

Body Scanning Relaxation/Meditation

This is a great technique to relax the whole body. It is best done lying down, but it is also fine to do it sitting upright in a chair.

In this meditation you need to draw on your consciousness and your attention to certain parts of your body. Imagine this awareness as a kind of ball of consciousness that you control with your mind. Start the process by doing a minute or so of breathing-focused meditation as described in the foregoing section. When you are comfortable enough, bring your consciousness to the top of your head. This consciousness is like a massage ball, and wherever you point it within your body, that body part automatically relaxes. As you start at the top of your body, imagine your forehead and facial muscles relaxing. Then move down to your jaw. Can you relax these muscles even more as you focus on them? Feel the tension in your forehead, cheekbones, and jaw just slip away.

Now focus your attention on the back of your head. The massage ball is moving around your shoulders—almost like getting a beautiful neck and shoulder massage—from one side to the other a few times. Now as you go to one side, let your attention move down your arm. Can you relax this arm any more? Feel it sinking deeper into the floor or your armchair as you focus your consciousness on it. Now come back up the arm, back over to the other shoulder, and down the other arm in the same way.

You get the picture. Go through your whole body like this, down the spinal cord and to the lower back. Move across both hips, feeling them relax more, and then down both legs and into the feet. Imagine it like a foot massage. Feel the tension in your feet being released.

Now work your way back up the body and imagine your whole body as the focus of your consciousness. Imagine your whole body now emanating a fantastic glow. Hold this for a little while, perhaps a minute or two. As you come out of this meditation, focus on your breathing again for a few breaths and then open your eyes. Aim to stay within this new relaxed state for as long as you can after you get up. If possible, don't rush up; relax into your day. This is also a great technique to use when you go to bed and prepare your body for a restful and rejuvenating sleep.

Mantras

Using a mantra-based meditation can be a profound way to focus your attention in meditation. The most common types are the om and the ahh meditations, although I would also suggest the Ho'oponopono prayer as a great mantra for meditation ("I'm sorry. Please forgive me. Thank you. I love you"). Alternatively, any text or prayer that you like can be used. Repeat it as you go into your meditation.

The ahh sound comes very naturally. In other words, it does not involve huge movements of your facial muscles. You simply drop your jaw slightly and rest your tongue as you let this sound come out. As you make the sound, focus on the noise being made. As always in meditation, if your mind wanders or thinks about something, don't worry; just bring your attention back to the meditation. The ahh sound is connected to God. In other words, the mantra comes from silence. It is oneness itself, and this oneness is God. If you can accept that God is omnipotent, then as you make this mantra sound, you connect to this timeless energy. You are in the company of God, and with each sound you make, you come one step closer to your Source, your Creator. Just bask in this knowledge as you go deeper into this mantra meditation. Make the ahh sound as you exhale, and for as long as you can with each breath, repeat the ahh as many times as you feel comfortable doing, aiming to get up past ten minutes with practice. This will leave you ready to face any challenges in your life.

I often use mantra-based meditation when I face any indecision or dilemma in my life, as it brings me closer to the Source. Often the answer I am looking for comes to me as a sign or a thought in the moments after practising this meditation. But it is important to state that I don't focus on the problem whilst in meditation. I just focus on the mantra.

The om meditation is the same process as the ahh meditation, but it is a good one to do in the evening or towards the end of the day as it can be practised as a gratitude mantra, giving thanks to your inner self, the universe, and your higher power for all that you have received that day, whether good or bad.

The Power Meditation (Super-Duper for Super Busy People)

Too busy to meditate? Well, if you are a super busy person in this super busy modern world with all its hyperdistractions, then this is all the more reason you should find time to meditate. You are the type of person who needs it most!

We often say, "I'm too busy." I think this kind of procrastination is really dangerous. It is that pesky ego again, stopping you from being your best self, causing you to remain in the comfort of the now nonserving habitual grooves that have been with you for so long.

Thus I give you an antidote. This meditation can take as little as one and a half minutes of your valuable time, so don't allow petty excuses to stop you any longer.

In essence, this meditation is based on the principle of a power nap. It's a practice that can fit in to your busy schedule and that you can do anywhere you can find a bit of privacy. Perhaps the work toilets aren't the nicest place in the world, but they will do.

Stand with your legs shoulder width apart, or sit with your back upright. Close your eyes and breathe in, counting silently to seven. You can count at a comfortable speed, not necessarily to the second. Once you get to seven, stop and hold your breath. Count again to seven, then exhale for the same count. As you reach seven on the exhale, stop and hold your breath again for a count of seven. This is one cycle. Start again and go through five or more cycles, as many as you have time for. Keep count on your fingertips. Five cycles should take about one and a half minutes.

That's it, you're done. A moment of peace in an otherwise hectic day.

Guided Meditation

Guided meditation is a great way to achieve a meditative state of greater depth by listening to a tutor and/or peaceful music. Allow the words and music to help you achieve your meditation, especially if you find it difficult to do so on your own steam. Many guided meditations are available online and are easily accessible. Of course there are many workshops and courses available if you would prefer going down this tutoring route to get the experience and meet like-minded people. I even have some friends who play guided meditations on their smartphones and listen to them with headphones on the train in to work, so whatever suits you, just give it a go and strengthen this essential spiritual muscle. I would say that meditation is nonnegotiable as you start to walk this walk.

It truly is your first step towards tuning into yourself, doing the internal work required to find yourself and transcend those old sabotaging habits, and creating new ways of living to move you towards your best and towards achieving your goals and desires.

In conclusion, start simply with breathing-focused meditation, and then let yourself be guided as to which path to follow. Personally I love, weather permitting, to meditate outdoors in a private space in my garden, or in my local park by a river, or under a magnificent tree. When I meditate, I often use the mindfulness method of bringing myself into the moment by tuning into the sounds around me. If I can do this outside to the sound of nature, then all the better. For me, there is something very peaceful in tuning into the sounds of nature. It helps me achieve a greater depth to my meditations. I also use the ahh meditation regularly, but I try not to do this one in open public spaces.

Smile Meditation

A great way to start your day, rather than getting straight on your smartphone and reading all the negative crap and bad news, is to try the smile meditation.

In fact it's an internal smile. Sit in position and close your eyes. Now smile to yourself internally. This may sound difficult, but actually, if you try it, you'll find that it is easy enough to do. You could also imagine a ball of light (like in the body scan) bringing light and healing to all your internal organs. Just follow it around your internal space as you go through the meditation. Try it on any injuries or ailments and see how much better you feel.

As mentioned previously, the mind is a powerful tool. By getting focused on your internal landscape, rather than straightaway getting involved in your day, you actually give yourself half a chance of being able to cope better.

Whatever works best for you, just go with it. This type of concentration and brain training is paramount to eliciting positive change in your life. Remember, start simply and slowly, doing only a few minutes, and then keep building it up. Aim to get to twenty minutes ideally twice a day, or if you prefer, a few two- to five-minute meditations. Meditating a little bit often is better than failing to meditate every day.

Goals and Desires

Getting clear about which direction you want your life to move in is really important. You can't reprogram your subconscious mind if you don't know what you really want.

Meditating and being more mindful, catching yourself in moments of being in autopilot, and bringing yourself back into the moment will be greatly beneficial to you. It will stop you from worrying so much, and it will prevent you from being concerned about what others think. But the greatest benefit is that this type of commitment to yourself will help you to get more in tune with your true nature, your essence.

As you do this, you can start to work out what it really is that you want out of life, what will really make you happy.

Maybe your number one goal is just that, to be happier. Perhaps you want to set up a business and be your own boss, having grown tired of working in the corporate world with which you are becoming more and more disillusioned.

There is a misconception that when one talks of being spiritual, it is wrong to want great abundance and material gain. This is incorrect because we already live in an abundant universe. If you are experiencing lack, then remember that, as you learnt in part 1, you create your experience. Your experience is linked to your thoughts and to your subconscious programming.

My life is not about making bundles of money, and my happiness doesn't depend on it, but I want you to know two important facts here:

1. I want to be involved with creative and fulfilling work that is aligned to my soul. I know that from doing this I will inevitably make money effortlessly. It's my birthright, as it is yours.
2. Personally, my happiness hangs on many things, such as family, having creative and fulfilling work, being fit, healthy, and lean, and being balanced and in control of my thoughts. Whilst money is not at the top of the list, I don't know any other resource as good as money that makes it possible for me to do a lot of the things I like to experience, such as travelling around the world and taking part in some of the sporting hobbies I have such as skiing.

Get it clear that if you are experiencing lack, then it's likely that you learnt at a young age to feel guilty about having any wealth. Perhaps you have inherited a poverty consciousness?

If so, don't fear. This is just a sign that earning more money should be on your list of goals. Make it your major desire to reprogram your life. Reprogram yourself to become a money magnet. Just think of all the good you could do if you were financially free!

If you are single, then it's likely that one of your major goals is to find your soul mate. Are you putting off going out to find people to date or meeting new people through dating apps? Have you lost confidence in your ability to find the right partner?

Often, these beliefs that we hold become self-perpetuating. As in all the foregoing examples, the only thing stopping you from having what you want is you yourself. Imagine that: you are actually impeding your own progress, basically by having the wrong beliefs and thus thinking all the wrong thoughts.

If you want more money but subconsciously feel guilty about having any, then you won't become rich. If you are single and want a partner but deep down don't believe in yourself, you expect someone else to.

It's not that I want you to feel bad about yourself; it's just I want you to go a bit deep here. Through your meditative practice, get honest with yourself about what it is you want from your life. Once you have done this, then *write it down!*

I keep a piece of paper in my wallet with the five main goals I have for my life. On one side of the paper I have written my base desires, which are to be happy and to have inner peace.

The goals I need to achieve in order to fulfil these basic desires are as follows:

- I am always centred and in control of my thoughts.
- I have completed the *Soul-Fit* book in time, and it is a Hay House bestseller.
- I have a beautiful and caring wife.
- I am bringing meditation to the masses, making it fun and accessible.
- I am a dependable, fun, and great dad, husband, and friend.

Notice that I have written my current life goals as if they have already happened. This helps my subconscious get to grips with them. The more I do this, the more I gravitate towards my goals. Also notice that writing *Soul-Fit* is one of my goals, so I'd better crack on and get writing.

I change my goals regularly, usually for one of two reasons:

1. I have achieved one of them. I'm sure when I do marry my beautiful and caring woman, she won't be best pleased if I keep that as a major goal!
2. Through the mental gym work I do, I decide that there is something else more in line with my truth. I get a new insight into the direction I should take in my life, and thus my goals need to be tweaked.

Life is a journey. It's your journey, so make it count. Don't stay stuck in old sabotaging ways just because you feel you can't change. I appreciate that leaving a well-paid comfortable job, for example, is not easy, particularly not if you have financial dependants and a mortgage, but if your job makes you sick to the stomach and unhappy, then why do that to yourself? You deserve better.

I can promise one thing: when you align with truth, when you find our true path, not only will you be supremely happy, but also the universe will conspire on your side. Coincidences, serendipities, being in the right place at the right time, and what will seem like magic will occur for you. But hold your horses. We are not there yet, so no making any knee-jerk decisions. When you truly know, you will know. You may have to stay where you are for now, but once you are in tune with yourself, you will instinctively know when to make life-changing decisions that will secure your success and happiness.

Once you have your first set of five goals and have written them down, make them your mantra. Meditate upon them daily, even if only for a few minutes, ideally in the morning and as you go to bed. If you find yourself on a train, take them out of your wallet and read through them. *Feel* the excitement of making these goals a reality.

Important Message

Okay, so making some goals and aligning yourself with your innermost desires is essential, but there is one rule here. Whatever you do, do not, under any circumstances, get involved with *how* these goals will become a reality. Do me a favour and leave that up to your subconscious mind. Remember, your subconscious mind is vastly more powerful than your conscious thinking. So don't even go there. So no thinking, *I will meet my partner at work. In fact, it must be the hot new secretary who has just joined us. I just know it's him [or her]!*

No, no, no! Whilst your new partner may turn out to be the hot new secretary, you actually are setting yourself up for a fall if you allow yourself to think in such specifics.

Allow things to happen naturally. Allow the universe to do its work. Your job is just to set your desires and move towards them. Meditate upon your goals for sure. Imagine yourself living the life of your dreams and *feel* how good it is, but under no circumstances should you get involved with how things will take shape, as that's not your role in this process.

Why?

Because you and I don't know the bigger picture. You may *think* that the new secretary is the woman of your dreams, but you hardly know her. She just started, right? Who's to say that the partner of your dreams is actually in the bookshop you happen to visit on a whim whilst on a weekend break to Devon. These things happen when you least expect them, so whilst I say to *dream big* and move in the direction of those dreams, I also say that you should have no expectations of *how* they will materialise.

What do I mean about moving in the direction of your dreams? Well, if it's financial freedom you want, then perhaps after a meditation session or perhaps whilst taking a shower after your meditation, you are hit with a moneymaking idea. Great! So you do some research, move in a direction. We are not thinking that this is going to make you an overnight millionaire (which would be getting involved in the how); we are just moving. Perhaps whilst you are researching that one idea, something else is presented to you, and from there a lucrative financial stream opens up. Maybe you try something and it fails, but you learn a valuable lesson, which means you are moving.

If you want to find love, you may receive inspiration to get on a certain app. Maybe you decide that attending a social event like a weekly pub quiz might be better. The more you move, the more you allow for the universe to present you with opportunities, meeting you with its side of the bargain.

If you are not getting the results you want, then look within. What's stopping you? What are the deeply held beliefs that are preventing you, and what positive programming can you do to help reset these beliefs? As always, the work is internal. It is within you and not anywhere outside of you.

Money will come to you when you allow it to; love will find you when you allow it to. You are a powerful magnet.

Like attracts like. You need to feel rich to attract money, and you need to love yourself and feel love to attract love!

In conclusion, set some goals. Don't worry if they're not perfect; you can always change them. But do become honest about what your true desires are.

Write your goals as if you already have achieved them. Keep the list short and sweet, including up to five goals.

As you become a more soul-fit person, your goals may change.

Meditate daily without an agenda (brain training), but once a day meditate on your goals, imagining your life once you've achieved them. You can do this a goal at a time or visualise your life with all of them achieved at the same time—whatever is most comfortable for you and most in tune with your desires.

If you can't get your imagination going, just read your goals to yourself a few times a day, feeling what it's like to have achieved them.

Resist thinking how these things might come to pass. By doing that, you'll not only limit yourself but also be thinking in a way in which they haven't happened. You want to convince your subconscious mind that they have already happened!

Neuroplasticity

A lot of what we are trying to do here with the soul fitness concept is to retrain the brain, to reprogram yourself in order to achieve success. If you are unhappy, then you are responsible for it. This is all about taking full responsibility and getting out of the blame game (i.e., looking to others and external events as the cause of your unhappiness).

Soul fitness is about working internally, getting fit *inside*. And as we have seen, the portal to internal fitness is the subconscious mind. The subconscious mind is responsible for all your habits, and it is a storehouse of memory. It's handy because without it you'd still be struggling to tie your shoelaces, and when eating you'd still be spilling the majority of food down your front. Oh, and you would be struggling to speak any language; thus you'd still be talking like a baby.

However, in addition to storing helpful behaviours, we also store bad ones, like binge eating and drinking, engaging in meaningless sex, and spending money unnecessarily. It's a dangerous thing when your subconscious mind makes a habitual groove out of a potentially harmful connection, like, say:

Finish work, then drink wine or beer, which relieves stress and creates a feeling of *happiness*. The happy endorphins are released because you have made that association, like Pavlov's dogs. The thought of that after-work beer or glass of wine makes the "saliva"— in this case happy chemicals called endorphins—whizz around the body.

We can see here how habits can form. These are neural grooves and pathways that obviously become stronger the more we repeat and reinforce them.

We can of course change them. We can create new grooves. In fact, we do so all the time, mostly unconsciously. Think about your commute to work. You might do it for several years, and then you change jobs to a different location. That first morning of your new job, if you're not careful, you find it would be very easy to jump on the old train going to your now old place of work. You might make that mistake once, but it's unlikely you would so again. Then after a week or so, the neural pathways have reset and you unconsciously jump on the new train.

This cutting and recutting of habitual grooves in the subconscious mind is called neuroplasticity, and you can use neuroplasticity to your advantage. The key is repetition. First you decide what it is you want as per the previous sections on goal setting, then you repeat the internal work to make it a reality.

This is where affirmations come in.

Affirmations

If I could get you to do one thing, it would be that after you're through reading *Soul-Fit*, even if you think it all to be a load of gibberish, you start and end your day with a repetition of the following, or any other positive affirmation:

Every day, in every way, I am getting better and better.

Say it a good thirty to fifty times when you get up in the morning and another fifty times when you go to bed, and just let it seep into your subconscious mind. Say it calmly and positively. Be as relaxed as possible. Regardless of what you think about spirituality, and regardless of what your situation is, just try this affirmation for at least three weeks in the way described and see the effect it has on your life, on your well-being, and on your outlook of life. Even after as short a time as a few weeks, I'll bet you'll see some positive results.

This particular affirmation comes from a French psychologist and physician who lived and worked over a hundred years ago called Émile Coué. Mr. Coué was a remarkable man. His methods, which involve mantra-like conscious autosuggestion, are designed, as he put it himself, to trick the mind. Just like what we discussed in part 1 when looking at the subconscious mind, Émile Coué knew of the power of the subconsciousness and positive suggestion. In his early work as a chemist, he noted how, when suggesting to patients the brilliance and efficiency of the drugs he was prescribing (even if these medicines were a placebo), this practice had a profound effect on the success of those patients compared to those to whom he said nothing. This is similar to what we now term the placebo effect. He was often giving just a placebo to those patients whom he told that the medicine was miraculous.

Mr. Coué then developed his methods with research into psychology and hypnotherapy. He also developed the above affirmation to help people overcome all sorts of maladies. This is called the Coué Method. For further insight into Mr. Coué and his work, check out his book *Self-Mastery through Conscious Autosuggestion*, which is a great read.

In essence, affirmations succeed because they allows one to focus the mind purely on the solution rather than the problem. If you spend all your time complaining of an ailment and all of its uncomfortable side effects, it follows that your subconscious, in tune with your body, will hang onto these discomforts, whereas if you focus on the polar opposite (the solution), you are far more likely to experience the relief of those symptoms. For example, if you have trouble sleeping, when you worry over it and build resentments, perhaps against your bed or partner who snores, you will likely, instead of getting your desired aim of falling asleep, become more awake. If, however, you find a way to release your resentments and worry and to focus on a sound and on restful sleep, then you will more likely fall asleep. If you will just repeat to yourself "I am falling asleep," over and over in a relaxed manner, you will likely slowly drift off. The paradox with autosuggestion is that if you try too hard or force things, you will probably get the opposite of what you want.

What do you do and say to yourself when you first wake up in the morning? Do you lie in bed for a while, checking your phone? Or perhaps you lie there for as long as possible, letting your mind wander onto all sorts of avenues, projecting about the day ahead. Well, by allowing the mind to wander like this, or worse still, project and worry about your day ahead, then you pretty much set yourself up for a bad day.

Daydreaming and imagination are not bad per se, but when was the last time you got up in the morning and really went to attack the day ahead with positive thoughts about doing positive and miraculous things? Because any great achievements in life started with a thought, as has been chronicled many times in this field, your thoughts are important, really important, so don't let them be controlled by an incorrectly wired subconscious mind. Start the day by setting the agenda and getting straight on top of your thoughts with positive affirmations and, perhaps, even by committing to an amazing miracle that you would like to manifest. Maybe today will be the day. By starting out in this way, you set yourself up for a much more positive experience. The law of attraction will make sure more positivity will occur for you. And if a challenge comes up (as they always do), you are in a better mindset to bat them out of the park, no drama.

The beginning and the end of each day is important. This is when the brain, as it comes out of and goes in to sleep, is in its slower wave states, alpha and theta. In fact, this is the state we can get into through meditation, which is why I say it's so important to do this type of brain training—because it enables you to reprogram your mind and consciously cocreate your own life. It's exciting, right? You can retrain and programme your brain like a computer programmer developing a new piece of software!

As our brains are in these slower wave states, they are more receptive to the aforementioned autosuggestion. This is where we can consciously suggest goals to the subconscious mind and request that they be achieved. It is during these wave states are that the subconscious mind will be its most receptive. Children, and particularly babies, coincidentally are pretty much in these slower wave states all the time. This is why we often say kids' minds are like sponges. It stands to reason, of course, that we have to learn a lot when we are in our infancy and childhood periods.

Thus, a word of caution. Because babies and children are so programmable at these young ages, particularly up to the age of five years, it is very important how we as parents conduct ourselves around them.

If you tend to put your kids down a lot, tell them off, or argue with your partner a lot in front of them, you are very likely to have a profoundly negative effect on their future. It's often at these young ages that children develop the insecurities, guilt, shame, and fear that can lead to low self-esteem, anxiety, and other issues that take many years in adulthood to overcome.

Remember I mentioned poverty consciousness earlier and talked about how it may have led to your not being able to accept or allow financial freedom? If this is the case for you, then it's likely that part of your parents' programming of you as a child involved them worrying over money and saying things like "Money doesn't grow on trees," "We have to work hard for our money, but there never seems enough," or "Life's so tough; money is such a worry." You get the picture.

The key to good affirmations, like goal setting, is to keep them short and sweet. Always start with "I am," and articulate only one goal per sentence.

For example, if your general goal is to be fit, lean, and healthy and always to make good food choices, it would be better to break that up into several affirmations, as follows:

- I am fit.
- I am lean.
- I am healthy.
- I, [insert name], always make good food choices.
- I, [insert name], am in control of my impulses.

You can also insert your name as in the last two examples above to make it more personal. The key is to write out your affirmations and always keep them simple. Ask yourself what would be the key affirmations to help you achieve your goals. Ask what it is that you want your subconscious mind to change or make habitual for you.

You can have a few affirmations for each goal. A great technique to help you repeat these affirmations is to write them on Post-it Notes and put them around your home or office, or keep them in relevant places, like by your bedside, so you see them all the time. Even if you don't read them directly but they are in your peripheral vision, your subconscious mind will still be able to pick them up. How cool is that?!

If you are unable to hang Post-it Notes all over your home because you are worried your partner and kids are going to think you've finally cracked, don't fear. Just write out your affirmations and read them once in the morning and once at night. If you can come to know them by heart, then when you do a five- or ten-minute meditation, use them as your mantra. If you have time, write out your affirmations daily on a new piece of paper—whatever works best for you.

They key is repetition. If you are unhappy with any aspect of your life, I can assure you that you have the power to change it. It's one of our gifts as conscious human beings. You need to throw the kitchen sink at it, though. It won't happen with you sitting on the sofa and praying for it all to change. Remember what I said: you have to meet the universe halfway. You have to do your bit down here on planet Earth. You must move in the direction of your dreams. Affirmations are a great way to do that.

Additional Techniques to Help Reaffirm Your Goals

Keep on keeping on. What follows are other techniques to help you continue repeating, and thus reaffirming, the affirmations and goals that you want to make stick. In doing these things, you will, without doubt, start to reshape the neural pathways in your brain, making it almost impossible for you to fail in your endeavours.

Ho'oponopono

Ho'oponopono is an ancient Hawaiian technique that has experienced a return to fame in the last couple of decades. I feel, considering today's times of great change, discontent, and material focus, that this no coincidence, as the practice carries a wonderful message of forgiveness, redemption, and hope, and faith that all that is, is as it should be, according to the universal grand design.

Ho'oponopono is based on the principle that we are all responsible for everything in our lives and that, as we have discussed in part 1, we interpret very little with our conscious realities. Therefore, by using this practice, we not only accept responsibility but also offer up a petition to the Divine Subconscious Mind for consideration and a remedy to our problems according to this divine order rather than our micromanaging of things with our inferior limitations.

The practice has its roots in group or tribal problem-solving. The ancient cultures from which ho'oponopono arose knew of the power of the subconscious mind and of divine power. The technique was brought up to date and made possible on a singular, rather than group, basis by Morrnah Simeona, born in Hawaii in 1913. Dr. Ihaleakala Hew Len is the chairman emeritus of the Foundation of I, the original centre for ho'oponopono studies and teaching based in Hawaii.

Ho'oponopono involves the repetition of four phrases—"I'm sorry," "Please forgive me," "Thank you," and "I love you"—which can be said in any order and about any problem. See some examples at the end of this subsection.

As with most spiritual practices, ho'oponopono involves the sense of a higher power. In this case the higher power is the connection between your inner self, your subconscious mind, and the Universal Divine Consciousness (higher power). You can still believe in God, but ho'oponopono does not support the idea of human beings being separate from God. Ho'oponopono teaches us that we are all connected and part of the some wondrous organism, including Mother Gaia (the Earth), the stars, and the universe as a whole. Ho'oponopono is also subject to twelve universal laws, including the laws of attraction and karma.

We can take any problem or issue in our lives, or someone else's life if we want, and direct our petitions to literally anything that we see in our lives as we learn that we are responsible for it all in the first place. It is, as per the law of attraction, happening to us, or in other words given to us by our subconscious programming, which is completely subjective, running on old memories, past traumas, and past programming. We might not like what we see in our lives, but we have to accept that we are responsible for it. It may even be bad karma from an old life that has come in the form of misfortune or a challenge to enable us to pay back that karmic debt. Through the ho'oponopono process, you can take this event, challenge, or problem, accept total responsibility for it, and show repentance ("I'm sorry. Please forgive me"), even if you don't know why the problem has turned up in your life. Just accept that you are not perfect and that you are subject to this subconscious negativity. Now show gratitude and love ("I love you. Thank you") for the problem, and trust that the Divine Consciousness will take care of your problem from its wider view, which is much greater than your limited view and much more competent than your micromanaging nature. Don't attach yourself to the outcome. Let go of the situation and just trust and believe that it will all work out for the best. Then watch the miracles happen.

Through proper practice of ho'oponopono, you cleanse your internal state so that it may manifest appropriately in your outer world. You are not attaching to anything but doing the work necessary—shortlisting what is not right in your life and saying the ho'oponopono mantra to seek the best possible outcome, the results of which can be mind-blowing. The point is to let go of your wrong thinking and of any resentment and get back to what is known as the zero point, the state of complete inner peace. It is when we reach zero that we can experience true intuition, as then we are not beset with negative energies like anger or resentment, which often lead us to make bad decisions.

The results of your petitions may not be as you expect, which is why I say don't expect anything. In fact, if you do expect anything, then expect nothing, as you will be blocking the process. Ho'oponopono is also about shifts in your perception. By practising ho'oponopono, you are living by sound spiritual virtues that say, *I am a responsible person. I live by principles of gratitude, even for the perceived bad things in my life, and I make love the bottom line in everything I do. Plus I have faith, utter faith, in the universal grand design of it all.*

In practice, ho'oponopono is very straightforward. You don't need a temple, a guru, a master, a church, or anything else other than yourself. As I have alluded to in *Soul-Fit* already, you are responsible solely for yourself in this life, for your thoughts and emotions, and you can have zero effect on other people's actions or the great scheme of things. This practice is between you and your internal world and the Universal Consciousness, so it is a great way for you to build your conscious contact with the universe.

It is meant as a cleansing practice. Ho'oponopono is a clearing of old memories and programmes that keep you stuck in negative patterns. With anything from addiction to an issue with a person or even a toothache, you can initiate this practice by taking responsibility for it, clearing your subconscious, and petitioning the Divine for a solution. You can also apply the ho'oponopono mantra to your goals and the things you want to change in your life as it is directly connected to your subconscious mind, the place where you are trying to build new habits.

If ho'oponopono does vibe with you and you want further information, then please visit the official website at https://www.self-i-dentity-through-hooponopono.com/.

> The Universe is a benign and loving place. … It doesn't want to hurt us. It's on our side. It wants us to learn our lessons. It wants us to succeed. It's up to us whether we do it the easy way or the hard way. It loves us so much that it won't ever violate our free will! It's our choice alone. … If we are deliberately making a conscious effort to resolve our karma, if we are trying to evolve, and going in the right direction, then fate will leave us alone to go our own way, at our own pace. … If the lesson has been learned then we don't need to repeat it.

—Paul Jackson, *Ho'oponopono Secrets*

Emotional Freedom Technique (EFT) / Tapping

This technique, first developed in the 1970s, is growing in popularity through the work of organisations like the Tapping Solution Foundation, which holds an annual tapping world summit.

EFT involves a simple technique of tapping softly with your fingers on selected meridian points on the body whilst saying your affirmations (of your choice) over and over until you intuitively come to stop, or as advised by a practitioner if you are using one.

It isn't a spiritual technique per se, but it has been adopted by many of the great spiritual teachers and writers, even by some of the more forward-thinking people in the medical profession, who all believe it should be used more frequently and as part of anyone's first aid kit.

Tapping can be used to deal with anything ranging from addiction, marriage problems, or money problems to big health issues like cancer or small pains in the body, physical, mental, and spiritual alike. It's also perfect. The reason I include it in *Soul-Fit* is for helping to instil new affirmations. This technique is great for that purpose because as you tap yourself, you can say anything you like. You can focus on any problem you have, so the technique encourages your subconscious mind to release negative energies and/or build new pathways. The tapping you do keeps you focused and centred on your affirmations or the ailments you want to treat. As we have seen with writing and repetition, heightened awareness or concentration on a wanted desire or goal is very much sought after in the process of reprogramming.

Tapping leads you to understand that any problem you have is essentially one you created. The process confirms that what we see in our reality is a reflection, a projection, generated from our internal computer, our mind in tune with our body and soul. Thus the best way—and this is the spiritual bit—to get over any problem is not to go out and find or do something outside of yourself but actually to do some work on and within yourself. Tapping helps release negative blocks and then recreates the reality that you want to see emerge as guided by your intuition. This is in essence what *Soul-Fit* is trying to get across, that whatever you desire exists in quantum fields of unending possibilities, but you must be the director of the process of grabbing it. You must set the script and reach out to get it. Tapping can help you do this.

For more information on tapping and the technique involved, please see check the following link. Tapping is, in any event, very easy to do. With some reading and perhaps a YouTube video or two, you can be tapping away in mere moments.

https://www.tappingsolutionfoundation.org/

Prayer

So maybe a bit of prayer can help too if you are that way inclined. Obviously to pray you definitely need a concept of a higher power. Otherwise, whom are you talking to?! Remember when I said to throw the kitchen sink at this? If you do have a concept of a higher power, then why not pray to ask for assistance in achieving the things that you want to achieve? However, please know that praying is not reading a Christmas list. You shouldn't actually ask for the things that you want to achieve; rather, you should ask for the strength and guidance needed to achieve them. After all, what is life without some challenges. Plus, do you actually want it all handed to you on a plate?

Never underestimate the power of prayer. As a wise man once said, "Leaving your home in the morning without having said your daily prayers is like leaving the house in the morning with no clothes on."

In his famous Sermon on the Mount, Jesus told us that God knows we need to be watered and fed and that we need clothes on our backs. Whatever era we happen to be living in, we have certain base requirements that need to be met, and our Creator knows this. Have you ever wanted for anything in this life? Have you experienced any synchronicities, lucky breaks, or "right time, right place" occurrences? I'll bet you have, as life has a way, no matter how off course we happen to be, of working things out for us. Sure, you might want to be driving a Porsche and living in a mansion with a sea view, married to Brad Pitt or Angelina Jolie or whomever floats your boat, but right now, you're stuck in Suckyville married to the coach potato of the year, you have a host of unhealthy habits, and you are driving a beat-up old banger instead of that Porsche. *But*, God or the universe hasn't let you down here. Rather, you have let yourself down.

You might be living an okay life. You might be married to an amazing person, or you may be single, living it up as only single people can do. You might have what is on paper a great job. But behind all of that, deep down, you are unhappy. You realise this unhappiness, though your half-hearted efforts to make some positive changes in your life seem futile at best. Again, who's to blame here, God, the universe, or *you*?

You see, your higher power has not left you to die of the insidious disease of a life in addiction or whilst unhappy amidst a seemingly endless struggle of mediocrity in Middle England. Not in the slightest. But have you ever actually asked the universe, God, or your version of a higher power for help out of the maelstrom in which you find yourself?

Probably, like most people, you have prayed for help when the chips were down, but let me explain that that is not praying. That is what we call begging, and when you are in that state of feeling super sorry for yourself, you can't expect miracles. All of a sudden you have gone from a disbelieving, nonpractising, cocky so-and-so to an overnight martyr who suddenly wants magic to happen for you. Sorry, but reality check—it doesn't work like that. You need to exercise your spiritual muscles, and prayer and meditation indeed fall under this rubric.

Build yourself a routine that works for you. There are no rights or wrongs in spirituality, as this is not religion. And it is certainly not a case of "Say ten Our Fathers and five Hail Marys" because you stole a hobknob biscuit from the communal work kitchen.

If you want to pray, however unnatural or silly it may seem to you at first, just find a quiet place and say a few words to yourself, to your inner world. It doesn't have to be poetry, but it does have to be heartfelt. The heart is the key. The heart is the portal through which you to communicate with your Creator.

Your higher power understands your words, but words are not the language of the spiritual world. We can say anything we want in our day-to-day lives. If we are honest with ourselves, we probably see that we lie all the time. Maybe we tell white lies, but it is dishonesty all the same. Flexing our spiritual muscles and changing our lives for the better is all about getting honest and being humble. As Mike Tyson, former world champion heavyweight boxer, once said, "If you're not humble, life will visit humbleness upon you." Prayer offers you the opportunity to be super honest and super humble. And by practising prayer, you start to bring these virtues into your daily existence. Once you are truly honest and humble with yourself, you become truly honest and humble towards others, which I believe is a key to living a happy and successful life.

May I remind you that your subconscious mind is a storehouse of memory? It records everything, absolutely everything, from the major events in your life to the most inconsequential thoughts. It is by cultivating more and more good and pure memories that you cultivate more and more naturally good and pure thoughts. These thoughts then become your reality. Prayer can play its part in this for you, if you want it to.

To sum up prayer, I would say that it is honest communication from the heart to the unseen. In prayer we can be totally honest with our Creator and with ourselves. You can't lie, because your higher power already knows all your lies and truths, and it's connected to your subconscious mind.

You don't need to make long lists of material possessions that you want in life. This is the universe you are praying to, not Father Christmas.

Ask your Creator to help you in your spiritual journey. If you don't know what you want to do in life, then ask God to use you. Through prayer we can hand ourselves over to the care of God. We are asking for God's will in our lives, asking to transcend our own will (ego-based fearfulness). Ask yourself, *Where has my will ever gotten me?* Are you happy now? Have things worked out as you wished? Through prayer we can hand our will back to God so that it becomes our will guided by God's will. In this way all our wildest dreams or better can become reality.

Don't limit yourself to what you might think you want in life right now—a Porsche, or a certain type of house, or a specific person as a life partner. These are all examples of self-will based in the material world. Use prayer to transcend these desires. Detach yourself from the hows and whys and whos. Become unconditional about your happiness. Try to see the good in everything you have in your life right now. Set some general life goals, like to live a happy, productive, and successful life, to come to know inner peace and serenity, to have a fulfilling and creative life purpose, to have an abundant lifestyle with complete financial security, and to meet your soul mate, and then pass these up to God through prayer in such a way that you programme your "GPS" with end goals and leave the finer details to your higher power. All you need to do then is enjoy the ride. Whatever comes onto your radar screen, accept it as God's will for you. Don't judge it; just live it. And most importantly, keep moving and be open to receiving.

Here are some examples of prayers that you can use, or you can just intuitively develop your own:

Prayers to Start the Day

> Universe, please guide me over the course of this new blessed day to be the best version of myself as I possibly can be as thy will is done. I ask that I may be open-minded and tolerant of whatever comes into my field of vision today and that any defects of my character and of my ego, with its judgements, self-seeking, selfishness, and negativity, be removed from my thinking. I ask that you give me the courage and

wisdom to see past my ego so that I may receive your divine inspiration and know your presence in all I do today. Amen.

O Divine Father, I know that you love me and care for me and that you give me all good things. I love you and think your thoughts and thus do only the things that you want me to do.

Prayer to Find Your True Significance in This Lifetime

O Divine Father, please use me. How can I best serve you?

I hand myself over to you completely now and ask that you guide me to find my true significance in this lifetime. I ask that I may be of service through this vocation and that it provide me with a fulfilling and creative existence so that I may be an inspiration to others, one who is able to demonstrate purpose, love, and compassion through work. Amen.

Prayer to Manifest Something

In prayer we can also appeal to the universe, to our higher selves, to manifest something in our lives. We can literally ask for anything as long as it relates to our true significance and as long as it serves the purpose of the Universal Subconscious Mind. I appreciate that this leaves a lot to the imagination, but a manifestation prayer should not be about a wish list. "Universe, please let me win the lottery" probably won't cut the mustard. Well, if you're the lucky one in three hundred million, then maybe it does work, but here is how a manifestation prayer relating to money or material gain might work:

Universe, please allow me the money I need to come from wherever it should come from and in the circumstances that best suit your divine order, as thy will be done.

You see, sometimes you need to take yourself out of the equation. Things always work out for a specific reason. They may not always suit you, but your time will come. As long as you remain positive, accepting things as they come with love as your bottom line, then the universe will respond in kind. Maybe one deal hasn't worked out only because a bigger, better deal is just around the corner. As soon as you start sending out negativity or resentment, perhaps because you believe your prayers are not being answered, you stop progressing. Negativity is the surest way to block your progression in life.

Prayer to Make Love Your Bottom Line

Dear God, I ask that love be my guide. I understand you to be love, the very essence of love, available and in abundance everywhere.

Please, Father, help me to see you in everything I do. I ask that I may make love the bottom line in all my dealings and connections today. Amen.

Prayer for the End of the Day

Universe, thank you for the day today. I pray to you now in appreciation for another day on planet Earth. I offer up these five pieces of gratitude for my experiences today:

[Then list off your five pieces of gratitude in as much or as little detail as you like.]

Amen.

Gratitude and Forgiveness

There is nothing more powerful in the spiritual realm than being able to show forgiveness. As Mahatma Gandhi put it, "Only strong people can forgive. Weak people do not show forgiveness."

Showing forgiveness is a portal into the realm of spirit. It is a human virtue that when practised can transport us to the fourth dimension. However, if we are to practise forgiveness properly, it must be applied to everything in our lives, not just when it suits us. And this last point is where a lot of us can fall down.

You see, true forgiveness is a sense of spirituality, a way of life. By blocking it, you also block the sunshine of the Spirit from your life. Not to forgive is to hold resentments, guilt, fear—all the negative emotions of the lower self that will keep you blocked off from your spiritual path and ultimately shut you out of your dreams, your goals, love, and happiness.

Perhaps that sounds a bit harsh. After all, we are only human and make mistakes, right? Right, but we need also to forgive ourselves, forgive the circumstances that might have created our wrongs, and forgive ourselves for all the self-harm brought on by being in unloving relationships or living out negative behavioural patterns. This is where forgiveness starts. We must accept that we are responsible for everything in our lives, including thoughts, behaviours, actions, and our past lives—the lot—and show forgiveness for it all.

We need to accept also that we are all connected and ascended from the same Source. The life force we all share is of our Creator, so we should not be judgemental towards each other. When you judge someone, you don't make an effective criticism; you only compound the problem that you are a judgmental person. So forgive yourself for any judgements you are about to make, and hand them over to your inner self, your higher power, for absolution.

To forgive is noble. There is nothing you cannot forgive in your life. Within this knowledge is the wisdom that everything is happening as it should, so by forgiving any obstacles in your path or perceived wrongs done to you, you are walking on the higher path.

In his book *It's All Mind*, Edwin Navarro writes a simplified philosophy of the famous *A Course in Miracles*. On forgiveness, as described in the course, Edwin explains that it has a different meaning from the normally used term and, as such, has an alternative, more spiritual meaning and practice for us in our daily lives. When used in the course, forgiveness refers to accepting that everything that we come across in our lives is a reflection of our inner selves. If we accept that our ego creates a lot of illusion to keep us in the belief of being separated from God—our source, all that is—then it follows that all perceived attacks, poverty, or general negative occurrences are illusions designed (if we allow them) by our ego to keep us in fear. It then follows that fear is an illusion (as God is love), so any events that we perceive as negative or fear based cannot actually be real. Therefore, rather than forgiving a person who may have attacked us physically or verbally, we actually forgive the situation or the *experience* of the attack and by extension forgive the perpetrator also. Furthermore, as our inner selves are the only part of us that know our true reality, our Holy Spirit (inner world reality) also knows the attack to be illusory, so we hand off all our resentments, guilt, and fears surrounding any perceived wrongdoing (committed against us or issuing from us) to our inner selves, to our Holy Spirit, and in so doing relinquish further power from our ego self and thus fuelling our ascension towards a better life.

It may be hard to accept such a notion, but I refer you to the opening section on keeping an open mind. It's also fair to say that this new notion of forgiveness does hold one bonus over the more direct version. For instance, in the foregoing example of being attacked, the normal style of forgiveness would be to specify that we forgive the person who has attacked us right? Yes, okay, we forgive a person who attacks us and then pat ourselves on the back for being a spiritually sound person. However, we are likely to then live in fear of further attack or the possibility of a similar attack occurring again.

This in effect means the ego has won as we remain living in fear. And if we are living in fear, we are not living on the spiritual plane and, as a result, continue to block the sunshine of the Spirit from our lives. To conclude on forgiveness, you can still forgive people directly, but it is much better to accept that you are responsible for everything that occurs in your conscious reality. When you do this, you can forgive and love it all. In doing so, you transcend the five senses, let go of any anger and resentments by handing it over to your higher power, and stop fighting with yourself. Let go and let God. Let go and enjoy your life. Let it all flow, let it all go, and end the otherwise endless struggle that you have been putting yourself through. Forgive it!

Gratitude

When I get up in the morning, I thank my bed for a good night's sleep! Think I'm crazy? Of course I am. In reality we all are. Who or what is normal? What we are programmed to believe in a normal existence is that the bullshit nine-to-five job is of value, that we should vote for some political puppet, and that all the crap of modern society is useful—*but this is not normal.* I hope you get where I am coming from by now, that you and I are unique, all seven billion of us. We are beautiful, amazing, and created in God's image, but somewhere along the line we have lost ourselves. So pull yourself together. *Wake up and be thankful.*

There is nothing you can't be thankful for. Showing gratitude is easy, and it is a spiritual cornerstone. In fact, it is a universal law.

A great way to show gratitude on a daily basis, thus making you stronger in this practice by exercising your gratitude muscle, is to make a list each night before you retire to bed of five things you are grateful for in the day you have just had, and chronicle these lists in a diary.

A change of perception is often required to be truly grateful because in modern society we tend to take so much for granted. We just expect things to happen, forgetting all the hard work that goes in to things. We have lost a sense of gratitude in our society and are now more prone to take to social media to complain or moan about things. A bit like the point made about forgiveness, if you are putting negativity out into the world, you are only portraying yourself as a negative person, so be more conscious of what you put out there.

Giving thanks and showing gratitude is a state of mind, a way of life. It is the ability for us, regardless of what happens to us (seeing as we don't have control over that), to see the blessings in everything around us, even the things that may see small. If your car breaks down, think, *Okay, this has happened, but I am grateful that I am still alive as this could have been a lot worse.* Refuse to see the negative side of life. Look deeply into any situation and you will always find a silver lining, blessings in disguise which you can be thankful for. And in this way you transcend the mundane, the ego-based thinking that will keep you pinned down in your old, negative ways.

Be grateful for everything in your life, and understand that if something has turned up in your life, it is for you. If it is a challenge, then rise to the challenge. Be thankful that this situation will be your teacher showing you how to become a stronger, better, and more thankful person. The Cantonese word for crisis is also the word for opportunity. Try to see the opportunity in everything that comes your way. Be thankful for it. Be thankful for the only thing in your life that you do have control over—your thinking— and make it count. Make it positive regardless of what happens. Keep practising your attitude of gratitude, and watch as your life becomes filled with things to be genuinely grateful for.

Physical Exercise

> We craft our spiritual strength through physical
> exercise, and our physical hardiness through mental
> practice—mens sana in corpore sano.

> Ryan Holiday, *The Obstacle Is the Way*

Good exercise is nonnegotiable given that the benefits are numerous.

The link between a healthy body, mind, and spirit has long been known, so it would seem to me that doing regular physical exercise is the easiest way to facilitate positive changes in your life. Anyone who exercises will know of the immediate benefits that are gained from working out. The uplifting of the spirit that can be felt afterwards can be quite addictive. However, what we want here is a sensible effort, not another addiction. And that is another well-known link—the replacement of one's addiction to substances with overexercising, and particularly the use of physical exercise as some sort of punishment, which is linked particularly to eating disorders.

Our physical, three-dimensional world is the easiest for us to interact with and have control over. Some of the other spiritual exercises and tools I have spoken about are harder to get a grasp of, and certainly entering in to the fourth dimension is not usually an overnight process. But physical exercise can be done at any level of intensity and in any place. You need not join an expensive gym or buy expensive gear and equipment. Just doing some light stretching each morning before you meditate would be a good start.

The great thing about exercise is that it can be anything to anyone. You only need to find something you enjoy and that works for you. So have a look around, try a few things, and see what you like on a trial-and-error basis. You might prefer a sport like tennis or netball as a means to exercise as this has the added benefit of a social group and also the motivation of playing in a team with others. You might hate that idea, so perhaps training on your own is preferable in a gym. Or just do some light jogging in a park. Perhaps you like long country walks. How about a martial art? At the heart of all the great martial arts are great spiritual principles and virtues that really enhance a person's inner world. I particularly like the art of tai chi, a practice that millions of people across the globe participate in each morning as a means of preparing positively and spiritually for the day ahead.

Good exercise is about having respect for yourself. It should be seen as a treat for your body. It is a treat to be able to give your body plenty of healthy exercise, good nutrition and water, flexibility, aerobic and anaerobic exercise, and ideally plenty of fresh air. If you can, exercise outdoors in a park rather than in an air-conditioned gym all the time.

It's easy to obsess about our bodies and how we look. We live in a world and society where image is everything. From an early age we are bombarded with advertising and glossy magazines, with TV shows that promote an endless search for perfection. Spirituality is not this. Instead, it is the detachment from this as much as is possible. Spiritually, exercising is having respect for yourself and freeing yourself from the prison of image and what other people think about you. You need to let go of that struggle, of that prison of perfection, because the more you seek outside of yourself in that way, the more you will ultimately fail. Why? Because the answers and solutions to the malady do not reside outside yourself; they lie within you. And physical exercise, done in the right way, is a great way of becoming more aware of oneself.

When you look at depictions of Buddha, say, the popular laughing Buddha statues, you always see what looks like a content facial expressions. These depictions are of somebody who looks to be at complete peace with himself. Images of Buddha are always a little on the plump side, with him in a comfortable position with his centre of gravity positioned low. Buddha is content because of the great realisation he had that all the happiness, peace, and serenity he had previously sought outside of himself actually resides within, and with that realisation came great understanding, great peace. It is the peace that you gain from ending your struggle, your battle, with yourself. He does not sweat a few extra pounds, his image, or what other people think of him, as he knows that to do so would just be a waste of energy.

Whether you believe in Buddha's teachings or not is not important. The lesson Buddha teaches us remains the same either way. His essence is all about finding your inner peace, not by attaching to material wealth and not on condition of anything, any person, any place, your image, or how you look to others. It is an inner peace derived from a letting go of all that and understanding who you truly are at your core. Your essence is the epitome of unconditional existence.

So with exercise, just get started, build it into your routine, let go of what your ego might tell you, and look within. If you feel silly, or if you tell yourself that you don't have time or don't have the energy, or whatever other excuses your ego may tell you to put you off, start to understand this ego of yours. Start to listen to your inner voice and intuition. What is it really telling you? The more you do this and the more you override your egotistical mind, the more power you will give to your consciousness and thus the more powerful and pure you will become.

Take back your power, exercise your spiritual muscles, and do some physical exercise!

Good exercise is nonnegotiable as the benefits are numerous, but keep in mind that good exercise means not overdoing it. That said, don't use this point as an excuse not to exercise. If you don't feel like exercising, then just simply commit to doing ten minutes. I can assure you, after going for ten minutes, you will carry on and end up doing thirty minutes or more. A body in motion is a body that wants to stay in motion, just like a body in rest is a body that wants to stay at rest (which is why it's so hard to get up early in the morning!).

Part 2 Conclusions

This section of *Soul-Fit* is all about building healthy habits and doing a bit of soul-searching to determine what it is that you really want to achieve in life.

Your success and happiness are guaranteed, though you might not see it that way yet. Understand that life is a great journey, so wherever you are on the path, you are moving in a general direction. Just make sure that direction is towards happiness.

Success and happiness are not the destination; they are the path and the journey.

Start cultivating some spiritual practices as outlined in part 2 of *Soul-Fit*. Through them you can start to reprogramme your life for the better.

Throw the kitchen sink at it. In other words, fully commit to your success and happiness, and you will make it happen.

Be clear about what you want to make happen. Make your goals your daily mantra.

Be grateful for what you have in your life *now*. You might not be where you want to be, but that has nothing to do with the fact that you will get there. And where you are now is an important part of the journey.

You need to fully accept and surrender to your higher self in order to progress. You don't need to believe in God, but it is helpful to have a concept of a higher power. You inner world can be your higher power.

The conscious mind thinks that it is making all the decisions, but behind the scenes the subconscious mind is really running the show. The subconscious mind is like a deeply entrenched road map that the conscious mind follows, not the other way around. You consciously make decisions and judgements and have thoughts based on the wiring of your subconscious mind, and this wiring was taken out of your hands as a child! You can rewire yourself, your neural pathways, to achieve, do, and be anything you want, but you must work at the sublevel.

You must go to the projector and not the canvas on which your life is playing out. The practices in part 2 of *Soul-Fit* will help you do this, whilst part 3 will enable you to make sense of it all and help you to make clear headway towards your desires, dreams, and goals.

3
Part

BALANCE

The Art of Balance

Leading a healthy, well-balanced, happy, good life is something most of us either wish to do or are actively trying to achieve. Leading such a life entails doing what you love, having a great partner, friends, and family, and having great wealth and success. Perhaps all this seems too good to be true.

Is it, though? Why is it that some people just seem to be more successful and happy than others? And what's their secret? Is it that some people are more worthy than others?

Hopefully by now you realise that this can't be true. We are all born equal, and we all have great potential. Sure, some people have tougher childhoods that set them back compared to those who are brought up with a silver spoon, but need I list all the overachievers in this world who had tough upbringings? The list is long indeed.

Regardless of your background and how much bad luck you feel you have been dealt, the basic fact is that you have all the power within you to achieve whatever it is that you want. The key component is you yourself. Your biggest challenge, your biggest competitor, in this world is you. The place to start working on achieving your goals is within you. It's not worrying about or comparing yourself to anybody else, as that is just a complete waste of time.

Get focused on your happiness, and be grateful for others when you see them living the life of their dreams—not your dreams, their dreams. Really, what has anybody else got to do with us? It's none of our business. One person's dreams are another person's poison …

Focus only on yourself. It's the only thing you can do. Don't do it in a selfish way, though. It's actually not a selfish thing. As you become happier, more successful, and better balanced, the more able you will become to be of use to others. You will become a better partner, friend, parent, and boss or worker.

True balance, health, wealth, success, and happiness are all cultivated from within. Through the practices in part 2 of *Soul-Fit*, particularly daily meditation, you can experience a more balanced existence. Having this balance becomes the foundation for your life, your health, your success, your happiness, and your true desires.

So what is true balance?

Well, I'll tell you what it is not. True balance is not swinging from one extreme to another like being on a roller coaster. You may achieving a balancing act, but it's not true balance.

Take going up and down in weight for example. I would know, as it's been one of my fairground rides for a big chunk of my adult life. It goes something like this:

I put on weight.

I look in the mirror and say, "Hmm, I'm putting on some weight. I'd better do something about this."

I don't do anything for a while, because, "It's not too bad. I've lost weight before, so I can do it easily again when I really need to."

I put on more weight.

Now I notice some clothes are getting tighter, and when I look in the mirror, it's, "I don't like what I see now. I definitely have to do something about this."

I go on a diet and start working out more.

I have a couple of slip-ups, and it takes way longer than last time, but I start to lose some weight.

Things gain momentum as I start to see results. I am back into your healthy habits and ways of living.

I feel good about myself again and swear that I won't let myself slip again as this was a real slog this time.

I start to become complacent. "It's fine. I can handle the extra calories. I never put on weight very easily!"

I put on weight, and the whole process repeats.

Time is a great healer. It's also a great magician, making it too easy to forget our vices. Drinking is another good one. How many times have you sworn yourself off alcohol, only to go a few days, weeks, or months without it, just enough time for you to forget how bad it was, and then start again?

This swinging from extremes may enable you to keep a decent average weight, but it's sure as hell a tough way to live your life. At some point, true balance will be much more preferable.

True balance then is about cultivating a healthy and good life. It's about being calm within so that when you face all the challenges and rigors of life, you are ready to handle them without falling back into old habits or swinging to extremes to handle them.

A balanced person is one who enjoys their life to the full, warts 'n' all. It's someone who is at peace with themselves, who doesn't need to prove anything to anyone, who would rather be kind than right. It's a person who knows the direction in which they are headed and that acts with integrity and humility. It's someone who is compassionate, first and foremost to themselves so that they can express this compassion to the world around them (because you can't give away what you don't have inside of yourself).

If you squeeze a grape, you get grape juice. If you rile an angry person, you get anger. And when you rile a compassionate person, you get compassion.

Who would you rather be?

Remember, being a balanced, kind, and compassionate person does not mean that you are a pushover or that you are flaky in any way. On the contrary, it means that you are far more focused on your goals and determined to reach them. It's just that you do this in such a way that it doesn't come at the cost of your own health or of other people's happiness. You are no longer on a rollercoaster but are on a train direct to your continued success, wealth, and happiness.

Unconditional Living

> The path with least resistance leads to crooked rivers and crooked men.
>
> —Henry David Thoreau

What conditions do you attach to your happiness, wealth, or success? Perhaps you will be happy one day, such as when you meet the partner of your dreams, or when you have sufficient money in your bank account or have the right job. Maybe your happiness, wealth, or success is linked to the condition of your environment.

In all these scenarios, there is one thing that doesn't change—*you*. Wherever you go and whatever you do, you are the root cause of all the perceived issues in your life. Let's face it: you are the one constant in your life. You are there from the beginning to the end and at all the bits in the middle. If you look at yourself now and are unhappy about any aspect of your life, then know that you alone are responsible for this unhappiness. If you are putting any conditions whatsoever on your happiness or any other bad habits you want to be rid of, then you are going to fight a long and painful battle with yourself.

The first key to true success and happiness is acceptance, and then comes unconditionally resetting your end goals. Once you accept that there are certain things that you are totally responsible for, such as your reactions, actions, thoughts, and behaviours, and then once you come to terms with the fact that you are completely unable to control the circumstances of life, other people, or your environment, then you will be living unconditionally.

It is such a relief to stop fighting with yourself, to let go and just accept things as they are. Life will always throw obstacles in your path. The path with least resistance is a terrible teacher. Furthermore, if you are choosing this path, what you are saying is that you want to just go from the beginning of your life to the end with no problems, no obstacles. Sounds pretty unnatural and boring to me. The universe has a way of putting the right things in front of us at the right times, as within each obstacle is a blessing. It may not be obvious to you, and you may not want to learn the lesson, but if you skip the obstacle, that is, by avoiding it and turning the other way, then you essentially move backwards in your life, having learnt nothing. By not turning up for life, you say to the universe, "Leave me alone. I want to go over here and stick my head in the sand and hope that when I come up for air, you will have gone and the path will be clear for me. Oh, and by the way, leave me some money and food before you depart!"

When you leave your dark hole, you will find that however bad things have become for you, the world has kept turning. Rich people have become richer, poor people poorer, and happy people happier. Can you let go? Let go of this fight with life and accept that things will not change unless you start turning up for life and facing your obstacles unconditionally. When you do this, it is the signal to the universe that you are ready to transcend your old self. And in that instant, the universe will set about to helping you. You might not like the type of help. It might be painful at first. But if you go about things unconditionally and with balance, then you will have a far greater chance of success as you attach no judgement on your route forward, taking each day, each moment, as it comes.

Imagine yourself in the workplace. Perhaps you are faced with a pile of work that you perceive to be impossible to get done in the time your boss has allotted for you to complete it. You look at the pile of work with resentment. How could your boss expect this of you? Your reaction to this situation is entirely up to you. No one can control your reaction to this situation but you. The pile of paperwork is going nowhere, your boss will be the same boss he or she has always been, and he or she will still expect the work to be done in the time he or she asked it to be done by. Those things will not change. So you have a choice. In fact you have several choices. You could allow the resentment to build. You could allow it to consume you, making your internal world a horrible place. And then guess what? As it is within, so it is without. Your time in that workplace and your day will just get worse and worse as you literally attract more and more things to get peeved off about.

Being unconditional about this situation starts with acceptance. You may then be able to adopt a more proactive attitude, which could entail approaching your boss and asking for more time and maybe involving a colleague whom you want to build a better relationship with. Perhaps this is the opportunity to have a heart-to-heart with your boss, or it may simply be the writing on the wall that you were looking for, the excuse to start looking for another job. Do you see the difference? Love your problems and love your obstacles because, in truth, that is the only appropriate response to absolutely everything and anything in life—compassion.

Present Moment Living

There is no better way to stay connected to your source and with your true significance than by staying in the moment. The present is the only time that there really is, as psychological time as we know it is an illusion. Yes, we need clocks to direct us through our working days, and we have the sunrise and sunset to tell us when to go to sleep and so on, but if you take all the clocks away and remove all the schedules and timetables, then what are you left with? I'll tell you: the answer is *now*. Now, this very moment, is the only time we really have, and in this very moment resides the beginning and ending of time, past, present, and future all rolled up into one. Can't get your head around that? I'm not surprised, because we have all been programmed since birth to see time as the standard linear cause-and-effect model that we all know and love. But it is merely an illusion as proved by Albert Einstein in his theory of special relativity and time dilation.

Whatever it is that you want to achieve, and wherever it is that you want to be in your life, you must first accept where you currently are. For example, see point B as where you want to go, the life of your dreams, and point A as where you are now, the present moment. Understand that point B arises from point A. It sort of bubbles up into existence through a series of life events that emanate from point A, from the present moment. Looking at it this way, you see that all of time is connected.

It is when we accept and surrender to the moment of now, to point A, that we are enabled to get to point B even quicker. It is by loving the moment and being at peace with yourself at point A, unconditionally, that you open up the opportunity to move in the direction of your most heartfelt desires.

I'm not as good at Einstein at algebra, but here's how it looks in an incredibly simple equation:

Point A (now) + Acceptance + Gratitude = Point B

Acts of Kindness

To perform an act of kindness may simply be to smile at a passer-by. It may be to help an old woman to cross the road. Or if you are feeling particularly joyful, you may even see to let someone bypass you in the queue at the supermarket or, God forbid, whilst you are queuing in the bank. You may decide to stop and give a homeless person some change or even give someone a $100 bill. The point is that as you activate the type of thinking related to how to be generous and kind, you start to overcome your own ego. You get out of your own selfish thinking and start to think more about your place in the world and how you can be of benefit to others. Always give unconditionally. If there is to be a condition placed upon this, let it be that you are trying to be a better person. Think that you are involved in the important pursuit of cultivating more balance and happiness in your own life so that you can be a better example for others.

Be Selfishly Selfless!

Get humble and see the connection that we all share in this life. As you cultivate your attitude of gratitude, also cultivate a sense of compassion for all things, starting with yourself.

Whom can you help today? Whose face can you put a smile on today? Whom can you seek to better understand, love, or console?

It's better to show compassion than to be right all the time. Let go of the need to win at all costs. This doesn't make you a weaker person, by the way. On the contrary, it will make you stronger. It will make your soul stronger at the cost of your ego. Conversely, any acts that strengthen the ego will be at the cost of your soul. So it's your choice: what sort of person do you want to be?

Acts of kindness are one of the surest ways to strengthen the soul. Just simple acts of compassion shown towards ourselves and each other are truly the food of the soul. Better yet, it needn't cost anything.

You can show gratitude to the shop assistant or the checkout assistant in the supermarket. You can open a door for someone. You can allow someone out when driving. You could donate some old clothes to charity. Whatever. Get creative with your acts of kindness. Where possible, make them anonymous and challenge yourself to do them daily. It will have a positively profound effect on your life.

Love thy neighbour as thyself, get out there, enjoy, love, and learn. Your story is far from over yet. Indeed, it's just beginning!

The Seven-Point Manifestation Technique

I did promise no three-point guides, but here's a seven-step guide to help you manifest things in your life. As you practise getting more soul-fit, the lines between the seen and the unseen will become blurred. The thoughts you have of things that you want to make happen will become easier and easier to implement. You will become the conscious cocreator of your own life.

For example, if you are having financial difficulties, the process to come out on the other side goes something like this:

1. Accept full responsibility, even for the thieves who stole £500 from your bank account the other day or for the bum deal that happened in your business last year. These things are all of your own doing as somewhere deep down you have accepted that somehow you are not worthy of financial freedom. There is guilt that comes from having wealth.

2. Show forgiveness for the situation that you are in, understanding that your incorrect thinking has brought you to a place of financial woe. Also show gratitude for the opportunity to change and for the desire to create wealth. You have some direction now.

3. Reprogramme your thoughts. Go within, meditate, use ho'oponopono, do some EFT, and use standard prayer and/or positive affirmations like "I am wealthy. I am rich beyond my wildest dreams, and money comes to me easily" or "I am becoming wealthy now. I will be debt-free by the end of this year, and I will have x amount in

my bank by …" If you like, write out your affirmation around fifteen times a day, as this will make it stick in the subconscious mind. Choose what you are most comfortable with. Keep it simple also. That is, don't utilise many different techniques. Use meditation and one other technique. Consistency is the key when looking to install new programmes on your hard drive.

4. Visualise yourself living the life of your dreams as a wealthy and happy person. Do this for a few minutes, a few times a day when you can, but especially at night before bed and when you get up in the morning.

5. Love yourself. Understand that this is your journey, that there is no good or bad, and that you will be provided for. The universe will make abundance happen for you if you allow it, so don't stress over it. Be patient and show gratitude and love for your situation, for what you will learn and experience. A resentment or any fear-based energy will block or slow the progress of your realising the magic.

6. Show gratitude. Be thankful for everything, particularly if some money does come your way, however small the amount. Visualise being thankful for large amounts of money too.

7. Show up for life. You are putting our clear intentions to the universe, but you can't expect things to be posted through the letter box whilst you laze on the sofa. Well, actually, this might be the way the universe works for you, but don't expect it to happen like that, because when you do, you are micromanage the how, which is ill-advised.

This type of process is flexible, by the way. The foregoing description is just the way I do it. But of course please feel free to make alterations that fit in with your way of being. One of my objectives when writing *Soul-Fit* was to make spirituality better understood and more accessible. When I have read other self-help books, I have noticed that there are always lots of points to follow and systems to use, many acronyms, and so forth. Whilst I think these are great tools, I didn't want to fill *Soul-Fit* with tons of information and exercises for you, as I know that most people who read self-help books, particularly hippie-dippie self-help books, are likely not even to finish any one book, let alone follow loads of protocols.

I wanted to keep the book simple, to make it a general guide. And then if anything were to resonate with the reader, they will be able to pursue that particular interest. When you open one door, it always leads to other doors to open, other options to select, and other avenues to go down. That is the beauty of life.

The foregoing manifestation technique draws on the law of attraction. This is a universal law that is open to all us—again, no exceptions. Of course some of us are better than others at utilising it. It takes practice and perseverance.

If things aren't going your way or you are not attracting what you want in your life, then look within. What is it within your thinking that is attracting the people and circumstances that fill your life? The great liberating fact is that if you don't like something, you can change it.

> If you change the way you look at things, the things you look at change.
>
> —Wayne Dyer

Unlocking True Potential

The potential is there; it always has been. As we grow up, we get overloaded with information and we learn many things. As we know, these learnings are recorded. Some help us and some don't. Learning to talk and tie up our shoelaces are things that are useful to us and make life a bit easier. In learning to cope with problems, self-medicating by drinking or taking drugs might work at first, but if developed into a habit, it can be very counterproductive in our lives.

As we go through our journey, the subconscious mind takes on more and more information, and without proper balance and a way of focusing the mind, we very easily go on autopilot all the time. We are not really living, just going through the motions. We are standing up with our shoes on with no clue, to put it bluntly.

It's fine to live like this, by the way. I did for many years and probably still do to a certain extent. The only issue is that I have noticed it. I have realised, had an awakening of sorts, that there is more to life than this. A journey of self-discovery lies ahead to reclaim more of my conscious reality. I may not achieve it in this lifetime. Perhaps I have too many obstacles in the way. But that's fine. At least I am moving in a direction and making steady progress.

In his book *As a Man Thinketh*, James Allen describes the mind like a garden. He says that when it is left untended, much like a common garden it becomes wild and unkempt. This is living on autopilot. When we start to do the inner work and start to tend and cultivate that garden, planting in it the seeds of change, the seeds of positivity, we set ourselves up for a great life. We may not always get what we want, but that's usually because we get something even better.

The mind can be a dark place, and there are many distractions, obstacles, and challenges for us on the way to our goals. There are a lot of obstacles in the mind that can block you from your true potential, but as I have alluded to previously, often these obstacles are truly the way. They signify the work that you need to do in order to unleash your greatness.

You may have heard the onion layer analogy or the story about the clay Buddha. These stories help you to realise that your true potential, success, and happiness lies deep within. You just need to undo all the wrong programming. You must uncover the layers of ego in order for this truth to shine. In essence, the light is already shining brightly; you need only uncover it. Some people have more layers/challenges than others, but remember, we are all on different journeys and paths. Don't worry about anybody else. Get yourself on the right path first.

When you are in the company of a truly balanced, happy, and successful person, someone who is truly at peace with themselves, kind, and compassionate, you will know it. It will be clear to you as this person's light will be shining from them. You will be able to feel the state of higher vibration that that person is in, and it's a great feeling to be around them. You are like this too. Show the world your truth and emanate this same eternal and timeless glow.

Happiness

Being happy is being content in your own skin. It's loving yourself so that you can be happy whether single or married, happy whether rich or poor, happy regardless of your outer circumstances. True happiness arrives when you realise that happiness does not and should not be reliant on outer circumstances. If you can grasp this concept, then you will be truly happy. This inner energy will allow you to attract all the circumstances to your life that you now know are not what makes you happy but that you nonetheless desire. This is the great paradox of true happiness: you will be happy whether you get them or not.

When you say, "This thing or that person will make me happy," or conversely, "The reason for my unhappiness is that thing or this person," then you are handing all of your power to the thing or the person or the situation. Take back your power! When you do this, you will truly be happy. You will become totally self-reliant, and in so doing you will be free to display your gift to the world. You won't need to worry about what others think, as you are no longer reliant on them to make you happy. This is when your true creativity can shine. It is when others will most respect you and look up to you, as having this energy will also be obvious to all. It will be admirable. This is part of your gift. By living your truth, being in balance, and being happy, you set an example to the world. This is how we each can do our bit for the universe, to repay the universe's love for us in kind.

A Fit Soul

To conclude *Soul-Fit*, I would like to summarize some of the key points made and theories proposed. I also offer you a suggested bibliography of books that I have found useful on my journey and that have been the source of a lot of the points I have made in *Soul-Fit*. Also, in the appendix are some other tools you may find helpful.

Souls come young and old. Have you ever come across a young person who seems beyond their years, not a snotty and annoying child who is extremely clever but terribly arrogant with it? No, I mean when you meet a young person who shows and displays great virtues such as love and compassion at a young age. This is an old soul in a young body, one who is on an elevated path. They are picking up from where they left off and are coming close to a life of enlightenment.

Younger souls make all the mistakes and live lives fuelled by fear. This is not a bad thing; it is just the way it is. I believe we must live many lifetimes to achieve the evolution that is the point of existence. For if not to grow, learn, experience, love, hate, fear, and all the rest of it, then what's the point of living?

I refer you back to the opening passages of *Soul-Fit*, where I ask, what is it that you really want, I mean truthfully, heartfelt, really? If you are reading *Soul-Fit*, then chances are you are on an elevated path. That you are seeking more truth is a sign that your consciousness is awakening. By practising the techniques to help unravel the mysteries that lie within you, you are becoming your true self—no longer a label, but the timeless warrior of existence that you truly are.

As you weaken the ego, you strengthen your soul. If you strengthen your ego, then you don't so much weaken your soul, but you prevent it from shining into your present reality. In this case, you will never, in my opinion, be truly happy.

Practice makes perfect. Daily meditation is a must. Keep it short and simple, and it is best to do it regularly. If you can get up to thirty minutes or more, then great, but just ten minutes twice a day would be brilliant. It really does help you to do the "gardening" of the mind. Meditation allows you to practise detaching from your thoughts. As you notice you are getting caught in your thoughts, bring your focus back to the breath, and just keep doing it, not getting upset if you keep thinking. Your mind doesn't stop thinking, so don't worry. As you practise, this extends into all areas of your life. You will notice that amidst the craziness and busyness of your modern lifestyle, you will be able to practise something similar. You can catch yourself when on autopilot and bring yourself back into the moment where, despite all the madness, you can still choose to be the witness, to be balanced.

When balanced, you are at peace. Your vibration raises. You are in a better state to handle all the challenges and obstacles that you face. You begin to let go of old resentments, and you no longer hold onto negative energies that otherwise prevent you from being the person you want to be.

Remember that when you judge others, gossip about others, or talk badly about others, you are only compounding the fact that you are not at ease with yourself. The issues lie within you and not the people you judge and berate.

Choose to be kind rather than right. It's these kind of behaviours that, as we cultivate them, allow us to become more successful at the most important thing there is to be successful at: being a good human being.

By cultivating a fit soul, you become a more humble person, a more loving, kind, and compassionate person. You can't give away what you don't have within yourself, so whatever it is that you want to give away, first cultivate it within yourself and let it emanate from you.

I'll leave you with this passage from a book called *The Instant Millionaire* by Mark Fisher:

> Live with this thought in mind: I refuse to die without having had the courage to do what I wanted to do. I do not want to die with the appalling thought that society tricked me, that it got the better of me and annihilated my dreams. You must not die with the dreadful feeling that your fears were stronger than your dreams and that you never discovered what you really enjoyed. You must know how to dare.

I dare you to live and accept the life of your dreams. You deserve it.

I wish you peace beyond all understanding. Love and light, my friends. It's all there is!

Appendix

Letter to Self

Write the following letter to yourself as you start on your journey of self-transformation. Write it as the guidelines suggest, and keep it somewhere safe, somewhere you can easily refer back to it and read it now and again. It will help you remain focused on what you are trying to achieve.

Take a piece of paper and address a letter to yourself in the normal way, starting with "Dear" followed by your first name.

Then use the following sentence starters and complete the thoughts. These will make up all the separate paragraphs of your letter to self:

I promise to ...

It's okay to ...

I am sorry for ...

You are powerful because …

I accept myself for …

I forgive myself for …

You overcame …

You have permission to …

You are allowed to tell …

I can trust you with …

You are capable of …

You can absolutely …

I love you for …

Apps and Diary Tech

'm a bit old school and prefer to use a handwritten diary. Each year in December I go and treat myself to a smart diary. In it, at the beginning where there are usually some pages to make notes, I write a review of the previous year's achievements with gratitude. Then, I write out what I want to achieve in the coming year. What goals do I want to achieve? Some are a continuation of bigger life goals, and some are new goals. We all change as we get older. New things come up of course.

I then break this down. Each week I write out which smaller subgoals I want to achieve. These might just be things I need to get done that week, for example, wash my car, and so this practice serves more as a reminder. Other things will relate to my wider goals, so maybe I'll include something like researching an e-commerce competition, which would relate to my goal of developing more streams of income. Then occasionally I'll throw something wild in, a real big dream. You never know! At least I'm challenging myself and the universe to make things happen. All miracles started as a thought.

These are the apps I use and some others I think could be useful:

Fat Secret – Calorie counter and weight/fitness tracker. I don't use it all year round, but when I decide I need to lose a few pounds, I find it helps keep me focused on my fitness goals. It's also good to use to see how many calories I am eating and how nutritious the food I eat is.

Law of Attraction – This app has many great free audios as well as e-books on the topic.

Duolingo – Great for learning a new language. Much better to spend downtime learning a new language than to procrastinate on social media.

Habitify – Another good one to load in some key goals and keep you focused on attaining them, this app is all about creating good, healthy habits that work for you.

Reminder function – I use my reminder function on my phone to message me every morning at nine o'clock with the affirmation "Every day and in every way I'm getting better and better." It helps to reinforce the affirmation and keep me focused.

Mind Space – This is great for guided meditations and audios.

Apart from these, there are thousands more, so just search and see what comes up. Another tool I use and think is great is the new subliminal software that you can install on your computer. If, like me, you spend a lot of time in front of a computer screen, this could be just the thing for you. The software flashes subliminal messages to you, ones that you programme of course, and it does this very quickly on your screen. Depending on the mode you set it to, the messages are either hardly visible or not visible at all. Get this: even if the message is not visible at all, the research shows that your subconscious mind still picks it up. Not only that, but also the message goes towards reprogramming your mind for the better.

Don't believe me? Well, advertisers have been doing this for years, and *it works*—big time! Companies spend thousands, millions even, on this type of technique to get us to spend our hard-earned cash. Reverse their programming with some of your own. Subliminal 360 is a great firm to use, and it's all very easy to set up.

Suggested Bibliography

Benner, J., *The Way Out* (Martino Publishing, 2010).

Benner, J., *The Impersonal Life* (Rough Draft Printing, 2015).

Carter, S., *Anthology*, i (Stuart Carter, 2018).

Dispenza, J., *Breaking the Habit of Being Yourself* (Hay House, 2012).

Dooley, M., *Manifesting Change* (Atria Paperback, 2010).

Dyer, W., *10 Secrets to Success and Inner Peace* (Hay House, 2006).

Dyer, W., *Being in Balance* (Hay House, 2006).

Fisher, M., *The Instant Millionaire* (New World Library, 2010).

Hamachek, D. E., *Encounters with the Self* (CBS College Publishing, 1987).

Holiday, R., *The Obstacle Is the Way* (Profile Books, 2015).

Jackson, P., *Ho'oponopono Secrets* (Amazon, 2014).

Jaminet, P., and S.-C. Jaminet, *Perfect Health Diet* (Scribe, 2013).

Jeffers, S., *End the Struggle and Dance with Life* (Hodder & Stoughton, 1996).

Klemmer, B., *The Compassionate Samurai* (Hay House, 2008).

Lefever, R., *Break Free from Addiction* (Carlton, 2003).

Lipton, B., *The Biology of Belief* (Hay House, 2005).

Madden, L., *Living a Safe Universe, Parts 1–3* (The Woodbridge Group, 2013).

McKenna, P., *Change Your Life in 7 Days* (Transworld Publishers, 2014).

Navarro, E., *It's All Mind* (Navarro Publishing, 2011).

Neill, M., *The Inside Out Revolution* (Hay House, 2013).

Shucman, H., *A Course in Miracles* (Foundation for Inner Peace, 1976).

Singer, M. A., *The Untethered Soul* (New Harbinger Publications, 2007).

Smith, C., *The Wonderful You: Your Purpose, Your Goals* (Hansib Publications, 2016).

Spencer, J., *Who Moved My Cheese?* (Ebury Publishing, 1999).

Titmuss, C., *Mindfulness for Everyday Living* (Bounty Books, 2014).

Tolle, E., *The Power of Now* (Hodder & Stoughton, 1999).

Vitalie, J., *Zero Limits* (John Wiley & Sons, 2009).

Williamson, M., *The Law of Divine Compensation* (HarperCollins, 2012).

Zukav, G., *The Seat of the Soul* (Rider, 1990).

About the Author

Well, first and foremost, my main qualification for writing *Soul-Fit* is the fact that I am a human being. I'm not a doctor or a professor, and I don't have a host of letters after my name. I am experienced in living and have found, through a spiritual awakening that I had about six years ago, that spirituality is for me and that it is a way out of most, if not all, of the maladies I am facing and have faced in my life.

I'm on a mission to bring meditation back to the masses, to make spiritual practice better understood, fun, and accessible, and to continue my own evolution towards whatever it is I'm heading to.

I am a qualified reiki practitioner, but I don't run a practice. If anyone asks, I am more than happy to oblige. I have done several distance healings for people, but I see reiki as a personal practice that helps me make a difference in the world by improving my own balance and connection, rather than a moneymaking entity.

I run a fitness blog and store online at www.EvolveandFit.com and a mindfulness blog and coaching business at www.JPRcoaching.com

If you want to connect with me for any reason, then please do:

Jacquespatrick.r@gmail.com

Lightning Source UK Ltd.
Milton Keynes UK
UKHW011813240419
341549UK00001B/26/P